Nature Through a Hospital Window

I0131790

Adopting an evidence-based approach, this book uses two state-of-the-art experimental studies to explore nature's therapeutic benefits in healthcare environments, emphasizing how windows and transparent spaces can strengthen people–nature interactions. High-quality, supportive, and patient-centred healthcare environments are a key priority for healthcare designers worldwide, with ageing populations creating a demand for remodeled and updated facilities. The first study demonstrates individual psychophysiological responses, moods, and preferences in simulated hospital waiting areas with different levels of visual access to nature through windows, while the second experiment uses cutting-edge immersive virtual reality techniques to explore how gardens and nature views impact people's spatial cognition, wayfinding behaviors, and experience when navigating hospitals. Through these studies and discussions drawing on architectural theory and history, the book highlights the important benefits of having access to nature from hospital interiors. This concise volume will appeal to academics and designers interested in therapeutic landscapes and healthcare architecture.

Shan Jiang is an Associate Professor of Landscape Architecture at the School of Design and Community Development, West Virginia University. She is also serving leadership roles in healthcare and therapeutic design for professional organizations, including the Council of Educators in Landscape Architecture (CELA) and the American Society of Landscape Architects (ASLA). Dr. Jiang was an AIA AAH Tuttle Fellow, Landscape Architecture Foundation Case Study Investigation (LAF-CSI) Fellow, and the Academy of Architecture for Health Foundation (AAHF) Research Fellow. Her primary research interests include the people–nature relationship, landscape design and human health, the application of biophilic principles to create supportive healthcare environments, and evidence-based design.

Health and the Built Environment
Series Editor: Mohammad Gharipour

Health and the Built Environment provides a transdisciplinary overview of community, design and health for practicing professionals and academics. Produced in a handy, accessible format and written by a range of leading international authors, this series will provide readers with a comprehensive understanding of the relationship between health and the environment. It will discuss key concepts such as restoration; healing and therapeutic environments; community health; integrated healthcare systems; evidence-based design; technology; city and public health; and sustainability, along with many more.

Urban Environments and Health in the Philippines
A Retrospective on Women Street Vendors and their Spaces
Mary Anne Alabanza Akers

For more information about this series, please visit: https://www.routledge.com/planning/series/HBE

Nature Through a Hospital Window

The Therapeutic Benefits of Landscape in Architectural Design

Shan Jiang

Routledge
Taylor & Francis Group

LONDON AND NEW YORK

First published 2022
by Routledge
2 Park Square, Milton Park, Abingdon, Oxon OX14 4RN

and by Routledge
605 Third Avenue, New York, NY 10158

Routledge is an imprint of the Taylor & Francis Group, an informa business

British Library Cataloguing-in-Publication Data
A catalogue record for this book is available from the British Library

Library of Congress Cataloging-in-Publication Data
A catalog record has been requested for this book

ISBN: 978-0-367-64105-4 (hbk)
ISBN: 978-0-367-64107-8 (pbk)
ISBN: 978-1-003-12218-0 (ebk)

DOI: 10.4324/9781003122180

Typeset in Times New Roman
by KnowledgeWorks Global Ltd.

This book is dedicated to my parents,
and Alyson and Yanwen Xiao

Contents

Figures

Tables

Acknowledgements

I would like to express my greatest gratitude to the people who supported me and inspired me while I was working on the research projects for this book: Stephen Verderber (University of Toronto), Matthew Powers (Clemson University), David Allison (Clemson University), Ellen Vincent (Clemson University), Ufuk Ersoy (Clemson University), and Andrew T. Duchowski (Clemson University).

I'm also immensely grateful to many colleagues, design professionals, and firms in support of my case studies and other parts of the book: Ali Dupnick/Perkins & Will; Austin Evert/HGA Architects and Engineers; Austin Ferguson/Heinle, Wischer und Partner; Benjamin Benschneider; Brad Feinknopf/OTTO; Bryan Dunn/Mahan Rykiel Associates; Diana Davis/Perkins & Will; Elizabeth O'Hara/Ratcliff; Emanouil Spassov/HGA Architects and Engineers; Emily Hagopian; Getty Research Institute; Hancheng Wang; James Steinkamp Photography; Jason Knauer/World Monuments Fund; Jennifer Sebranek/GBBN; Jim Keller/SiteWorkshop; Kalpana Kuttaiah/Perkins & Will; Julia Leitman/ZGF; Katie Simpson/ Perkins & Will; Kirsten Miller/GBBN; Lasse Tur; Laura Crawford/ Perkins & Will; Lauren Hunt/SAGE Publishing; Lorenz Siegenthaler/ August + Margrith Künzel Landschaftsarchitekten AG; Maaike van der Velden/BiermanHenket; Maria Gertell/White Arkitekter; Matthew Wood/ SiteWorkshop; Megan Barnes/Landscape Architecture Foundation; Michael Haas/GBBN; Michel Kievits/Sybolt Voeten; Minglu Lin/Perkins & Will; Mladena Žarković/Studio 3LHD; Nikken Sekkei Ltd.; Reuben M. Rainey/University of Virginia; Scott Abernethy/ZGF; Tim Griffith; Todd Kohli/Smith Group, and Yanwen Xiao.

Additionally, my special thanks are addressed to my research assistants from West Virginia University, Udday Datta, Noah Cremeans, Mariami Maghlakelidze, Sofija Kaljevic, Debsree Mandal, and Yasmeen Mohammed Ali, who have helped me in different phases of the projects for this book. I also own a special thanks to my colleagues at the School of Design and Community Development, West Virginia University, who covered my duties during my sabbatical leave for this book.

The projects in this book would not have been possible without the sponsor of the following funding agencies: Academy of Architecture for Health Foundation Research Grant, Landscape Architecture Foundation Case Study Investigation Program (LAF CSI), AIA AAH Arthur N. Tuttle Jr. Graduate Fellowship, West Virginia Agricultural and Forestry Experiment Station Fund, HATCH Grant, and Daniel C. & Elizabeth D. Brown Faculty Development Fund and Kaye C. Daniel Faculty Development Award provided by the Davis College of Agricultural, Natural Resources and Design at West Virginia University.

1 Introduction

High-quality, supportive, and patient-centered healthcare environments remain the top focus of healthcare designers worldwide. The aging population globally (United Nations, 2019) has created a demand for remodeled and updated healthcare facilities, and the COVID-19 pandemic revealed the shortage of healthcare resource and disparate medical coverage in many regions around the world (Blumenthal et al., 2020). Therefore, the construction of new healthcare facilities and the reshaping of existing ones will be a growing trend in the US and throughout the world (Morgan & Burmahl, 2021). Large hospitals, particularly those influenced by modernism architecture, have been criticized for their ignorance of humanistic concerns in many ways, including the deprivation of therapeutic contact with nature and inadequate greenspaces on campus that are visually and physically accessible (Cooper Marcus, 2007; Verderber, 2006). In fact, such a highly institutional environment is itself accountable for many stressful conditions and negative outcomes that occupants acquire in the hospital (Ulrich, 2001; Ulrich et al., 2004). Since the rise of evidence-based design (EBD) in correspondence to patient-centered care in the 1990s, accumulating evidence has proven the benefits of the humanized healthcare environment, among which nature and hospital greenspaces were found to play important roles in restoring people from stress and fatigue, and facilitating patient recovery from medical treatments (Cooper Marcus & Barnes, 1999; Cooper Marcus & Sachs, 2013; Cordoza et al., 2018; Moore, 2007; Ulrich, 1984).

People interact with nature in hospitals through two forms: through windows and visual contact with nature or by physically being present in a greenspace. Either form of nature interaction reminds the existence of a clear boundary between the inside and outside domains in the hospital. Patients with limited mobility mostly rely on the former type of interaction with nature, looking out to the outside through a small window in their patient rooms. Gardens and natural features that are disconnected from the hospital building require extensive effort to visit from a patient room as one must travel through labyrinthine corridors and multiple transitions between departmental units until arriving outside. Even staff members who are mobile have reported the long traveling distance as a factor impeding

DOI: 10.4324/9781003122180-1

their use of many greenspaces on a large medical campus (Jiang & Kaljevic, 2017). Low visibility and accessibility, as well as the disconnected indoor–outdoor relationship, hinder the effective people–nature interactions in hospital environments. Therefore, it is necessary to reinvent the relationship among the site, landscape, and building by "dematerializing the physical and symbolic barriers that cut the interior of a building off from the outside world" so that nature's therapeutic benefits can be revealed and the hospital building can breathe (Verderber, 2010, p. 52).

Scope and Key Concepts

Adopting an evidence-based approach while employing multiple research perspectives and methods, this book discusses the therapeutic benefits of nature and landscapes in healthcare architectural design. The emphases of this book lie on people–nature interactions through windows, transparency, and transitions between the inside and outside environments in the public spaces of large healthcare facilities. The design for patient rooms and private spaces in which patients receive treatment and operations is not the emphasis of the book. In addition, the book does not address gardening, rehabilitative activities, or nature-based therapeutic interventions as defined by the professions of horticultural therapy and occupational therapy (American Horticultural Therapy Association, n.d.; Stigsdotter et al., 2010). Some essential concepts that repeat throughout the book are explained here to facilitate understanding of the texts.

EBD is the established framework for the content of this book. The Center for Health Design (n.d.) defined EBD as "the process of basing decisions about the built environment on credible research to achieve the best possible outcomes." The design for any type of healthcare environment should follow rigorous steps that include collecting and critically interpreting relevant evidence, developing a hypothesis and testing it through research studies, collecting baseline performance measures, and conducting a post-occupancy evaluation (POE) of the design (The Center for Health Design, n.d.). EBD has been considered effective in making healthcare planning and design decisions that benefit key stakeholders and achieve the best patient, staff, and operational outcomes, including but not limited to the audio and visual environment, safety enhancement, wayfinding system, sustainability, patient room, and spaces that support family, staff, and physicians in healthcare facilities (Ulrich et al., 2010).

In order to explain the healing effect of nature, several concepts—often used interchangeably—have been employed in this book. The term "therapeutic landscapes" was first introduced by medical geographers to explore why certain places with natural or historic features have an enduring reputation for the maintenance of health and well-being (Bell et al., 2018; Gesler, 1992, 2003). Hickman (2013) defined therapeutic landscapes as the immediate gardens and wider open spaces that can be accessed or viewed from institutions whose primary concern is related to medical practice. Parallelly, the term "restorative environment" or "nature restoration" originates from Kaplan and Kaplan's (1989) studies of people's experiences of nature in the wildness, leading to the exploration of nature's restorative effects in mental fatigue relief. Several arenas of research converge (as discussed in Chapter 2) and the therapeutic/restorative concepts have been evolving and expanding, often being used interchangeably, to represent a wide range of greenspaces designed to offer health benefits (Cooper Marcus & Sachs, 2013; Gerlach-Spriggs et al., 1998; Tyson, 1998). The current book interchangeably refers to "therapeutic landscapes" and "nature restoration" as umbrella terms for a wide range of natural settings that improve people's physical, psychological, emotional, spiritual, and social well-being.

In the seminal edition of *Healing Gardens* (Cooper Marcus & Barnes, 1999), the term "healing garden" was systematically discussed as referring to a variety of garden features that "foster restoration from stress and have other positive influences on patients, visitors, and staff or caregivers" (Ulrich, 1999, p. 30). The term "healing garden" has also been adapted to a wider range of meanings in subsequent scholarship, being used interchangeably with "hospital garden," "therapeutic garden," and "restorative outdoor spaces" in the medical context (Cooper Marcus & Sachs, 2013; Helphand, 2019). The current book uses "hospital greenspaces" as an umbrella term to represent any indoor or outdoor spaces that integrate plants and natural materials as the predominant features in a large healthcare facility.

Organization

The book unfolds the examination of nature's therapeutic effects from an overview of the history and theory of nature restoration and people–nature interaction through windows. Adopting an evidence-based approach, the core of the book consists of two state-of-the-art experimental studies to explore nature's therapeutic benefits in large healthcare facilities, emphasizing how windows and transparent spaces can strengthen people–nature interactions. The first experiment tested people's psychophysiological responses, moods, and preferences in simulated hospital waiting areas with different levels of visual access to nature through windows and transparency. The second experiment employed cutting-edge immersive virtual reality techniques to explore how gardens and daylight impact people's spatial cognition, wayfinding behaviors, and experience when navigating hospitals.

Chapter 2 demonstrates the breadth, depth, and multifacetedness of the topics of nature restoration through cross-disciplinary lenses, including cultural and historical perspectives, medical geography, evolutional perspectives, environmental psychology and behavioral studies, and public health. It also examines nature's therapeutic effects and the underlying healing mechanisms through a closer review of some dominant schools of thoughts, highlighting the attention-restoration theory (Kaplan & Kaplan, 1989), stress reduction theory (Ulrich, 1983), and integrative framework of both (Kaplan, 1995).

Chapter 3 reviews the importance of windows in various built environments as a primary means and micro-restorative settings that provide a connection between occupants and the external world. A series of window attributes are discussed with regard to occupants' preferences and the health benefits. The presence of window views of nature and natural daylight and their therapeutic effects on patients and staff members are discussed in greater depth, indicating the imperativeness of establishing a connection between people and the outside nature through windows in healthcare environments.

Chapter 4 explores the ascending/declining dynamics of the people–nature relationship in hospitals through an expedited review of the hospital design in modern and contemporary history. Lessons learned from the tuberculosis sanatorium movement between the two world wars are documented, with a particular emphasis on the windows, indoor–outdoor transition, and greenspaces in the sanatoriums. The revival of greenspaces in contemporary hospitals is also discussed, with some prominent usage issues identified. Two recent POE studies (Jiang et al., 2018) examined different hospital greenspaces and concluded that the locations of the greenspaces as well as the spatial relationship to the medical buildings affect the usage of the greenspaces in a hospital environment.

Chapter 5 raises a concern that contemporary hospital design should deconstruct the condensed, mega-building blocks and introduce nature, pleasant views, and daylight through *theraserialization* (Verderber, 2010). This chapter follows the initial theories of literal and phenomenal transparency by Rowe and Slutzky (1963), then further expands Hoesli's (1997) claim that phenomenal transparency stands as a method of perception as well as a design tool that handles the spatial continuity issues of architectural spaces. Phenomenal transparency generates in-between spaces that blur building boundaries and form a spatial continuum that interrelates built and natural environments. A preliminary pattern language of transparent spaces is proposed as summarized from Alexander and colleagues' (1977) typological study of buildings, towns, and constructions. The 12 patterns of transparency design are elaborated through 34 contemporary cases in the case study chapter (Chapter 8) in order to strengthen the indoor–outdoor connectivity on a medical campus or in a large hospital building.

Chapter 6 sheds light on implementing therapeutic landscape-viewing patterns in the design of waiting areas and other healthcare interior spaces with seating opportunities. A quasi-experimental study is detailed, including all essential components in the process of a systematic inquiry, which serves as an example in planning similar studies in the realm. Additional findings from recent empirical studies about healthcare waiting experience and the related spatial design issues are translated into applicable design suggestions to indicate future practices. The static and in-motion statuses compose the two fundamental types of experiences between humans and their environment. People's kinetic experience in healthcare environments is associated with their spatial cognitive process and wayfinding behaviors to a great extent. Whereas Chapter 6 discusses people's waiting experience—a commonly static status during healthcare—and the design applications of the pattern therapeutic viewing places, Chapter 7 focuses on the "transparent arteries" pattern and explores how the inside-out transition, window views of nature and daylight, and transparency attributes impact people's experiences and behaviors in motion. The findings from recent empirical studies about healthcare wayfinding experiences and the related spatial design issues are translated into applicable design suggestions for future practices.

Two major behaviors in healthcare public spaces—waiting and wayfinding—affect people's perceptions of hospital design and perceived quality of care. This book documents new knowledge about nature's therapeutic benefits in waiting and circulation areas, highlighting the importance of having access to nature from hospital interiors. The theoretical discussion of architectural theory, including literal and phenomenal transparency, reappraises the design of healthcare's public areas to promote the continuum between architecture and therapeutic landscapes. The research protocols apply to explorations in environmental psychology, behavior, and cognition, as well as architectural and landscape architectural design in healthcare. The book concludes the discussion in Chapter 9, suggesting that paradigms of hospital environment design are shifting and offering some forward-looking thoughts regarding the future trends of hospital greenspaces in the wake of the COVID-19 pandemic.

References

Alexander, C., Ishikawa, S., Silverstein, M., Jacobson, M., Fiksdahl-King, I., & Angel, S. (1977). *A pattern language: Towns, buildings, construction.* Oxford University Press.

American Horticultural Therapy Association. (n.d.). *About therapeutic gardens: A word about therapeutic gardens.* https://www.ahta.org/about-therapeutic-gardens

Bell, S. L., Foley, R., Houghton, F., Maddrell, A., & Williams, A. M. (2018). From therapeutic landscapes to healthy spaces, places and practices: A scoping review. *Social Science & Medicine, 196,* 123–130.

Blumenthal, D., Fowler, E. J., Abrams, M., & Collins, S. R. (2020, October 8). Covid-19—Implications for the health care system. *The New England Journal of Medicine, 383,* 1483–1488. 10.1056/NEJMsb2021088

Cooper Marcus, C. (2007). Healing gardens in hospitals. *Interdisciplinary Design and Research E-Journal, 1*(1).

Cooper Marcus, C., & Barnes, M. (Eds.). (1999). *Healing gardens: Therapeutic benefits and design recommendations.* Wiley.

Cooper Marcus, C., & Sachs, N. A. (2013). *Therapeutic landscapes: An evidence-based approach to designing healing gardens and restorative outdoor spaces.* John Wiley & Sons.

Cordoza, M., Ulrich, R. S., Manulik, B. J., Gardiner, S. K., Fitzpatrick, P. S., Hazen, T. M., Mirka, A., & Perkins, R. S. (2018). Impact of nurses taking daily work breaks in a hospital garden on burnout. *American Journal of Critical Care, 27*(6), 508–512.

Gerlach-Spriggs, N., Kaufman, R. E., & Warner, S. B. (1998). *Restorative gardens: The healing landscape.* Yale University Press.

Gesler, W. M. (1992). Therapeutic landscapes: Medical issues in light of the new cultural geography. *Social Science & Medicine, 34*(7), 735–746.

Gesler, W. M. (2003). *Healing places.* Rowman & Littlefield.

Helphand, K. I. (2019). Prescribing the outdoors: A model hospital garden. *Site/LINES Fall 2019: Designing for Wellness: Therapeutic Landscapes, 9*(1), 10–12.

Hickman, C. (2013). *Therapeutic landscapes: A history of English hospital gardens since 1800.* Manchester University Press.

Hoesli, B. (1997). Transparent form-organization as an instrument of design. In C. Rowe, R. Slutzky, & B. Hoesli (Eds.), *Transparency.* Birkhauser.

Jiang, S., & Kaljevic, S. (2017). *Owensboro health regional hospital. Landscape performance series.* Landscape Architecture Foundation. https://doi.org/10.31353/cs1211

Jiang, S., Staloch, K., & Kaljevic, S. (2018). Opportunities and barriers to using hospital gardens: Comparative post occupancy evaluations of healthcare landscape environments. *Journal of Therapeutic Horticulture, 28*(2), 23–56.

Kaplan, R., & Kaplan, S. (1989). *The experience of nature: A psychological perspective.* CUP Archive.

Kaplan, S. (1995). The restorative benefits of nature: Toward an integrative framework. *Journal of Environmental Psychology, 15*(3), 169–182.

Moore, K. D. (2007). Restorative dementia gardens: Exploring how design may ameliorate attention fatigue. *Journal of Housing for the Elderly, 21*(1–2), 73–88.

Morgan, J., & Burmahl, B. (2021, April 22). 2021 hospital construction survey: Hospitals and contractors take on pandemic-related building and design challenges. *Health Facilities Management.* https://www.hfmmagazine.com/articles/4148-2021-hospital-construction-survey

Rowe, C., & Slutzky, R. (1963). Transparency: Literal and phenomenal. *Perspecta, 8*, 45–54.

Stigsdotter, U. K., Palsdottir, A. M., Burls, A., Chermaz, A., Ferrini, F., & Grahn, P. (2010). Nature-based therapeutic interventions. In K. Nilsson, M. Sangster, C. Gallis, T. Hartig, S. de Vries, K. Seeland, & J. Schipperijn (Eds.), *Forests, trees and human health* (pp. 309–342). Springer.

The Center for Health Design. (n.d.). *About EBD: What is evidence-based design (EBD)?.* https://www.healthdesign.org/certification-outreach/edac/about-ebd

Tyson, M. M. (1998). *The healing landscape: Therapeutic outdoor environments.* McGraw-Hill.

Ulrich, R. S. (1983). Aesthetic and affective response to natural environment. In I. Altman & J. F. Wohlwill (Eds.), *Human behavior and environment: Advances in theory and research* (Vol. 6; pp. 85–125). Plenum.

Ulrich, R. S. (1984). View through a window may influence recovery from surgery. *Science, 224*(4647), 420–421.

Ulrich, R. S. (1999). Effects of gardens on health outcomes: Theory and research. In C. Cooper Marcus, & M. Barnes (Eds.), *Healing gardens: Therapeutic benefits and design recommendations* (pp. 27–86). Wiley.

Ulrich, R. S. (2001). Effects of healthcare environmental design on medical outcomes. *Design and health: Proceedings of the Second International Conference on Health and Design*, 49, 49–59.

Ulrich, R. S., Berry, L. L., Quan, X., & Parish, J. T. (2010). A conceptual framework for the domain of evidence-based design. *Health Environments Research & Design Journal*, 4(1), 95–114.

Ulrich, R. S., Quan, X., Zimring, C., Joseph, A., & Choudhary, R. (2004, September). The role of the physical environment in the hospital of the 21st century: A once-in-a-lifetime opportunity. *The Center for Health Design*. https://www.healthdesign.org/knowledge-repository/role-physical-environment-hospital-21st-century-once-lifetime-opportunity

United Nations, Department of Economic and Social Affairs, Population Division. (2019). *World population prospects 2019: Highlights* (ST/ESA/SER.A/423). https://population.un.org/wpp/Publications/Files/WPP2019_Highlights.pdf

Verderber, S. (2006). Hospital futures—humanism versus the machine. In C. Wagenaar (Ed.), *The architecture of hospitals* (pp. 76–87). NAi Publishers

Verderber, S. (2010). *Innovations in hospital architecture*. Routledge.

2 The History and Theory of Nature's Therapeutic Effects

In the history of human development, nature has traditionally been viewed as a "healer." Almost every culture includes the concept of paradise as a garden, in which plants, water, and a variety of natural elements are perceived as sacred symbols of healing (Squire, 2002). Ranging from the individual elements to the holistic relationship between people and the environment, from ancient beliefs to recent scientific findings, nature contains numerous facets that can be interpreted as therapeutic. This chapter first highlights several cultural and historical examples that demonstrate nature's therapeutic effects and then reviews the contemporary theories that explain why and how nature can heal.

The Traditional Belief that Nature Heals

Air, Water, and Places

Hippocrates (460–377 BCE), the ancient Greek physician and founder of science-based medicine, elaborated on the importance of environmental factors in the practice of medicine in his book *On Airs, Waters, and Places*:

> Whoever wishes to investigate medicine properly, should proceed thus: in the first place to consider the seasons of the year … then the winds, the hot and the cold …. We must also consider the qualities of the waters … when one comes into a city to which he is a stranger, he ought to consider its situation, how it lies as to the winds and the rising of the sun. (Hippocrates, 2010, p. 3)

In similar manner, ancient Chinese followed *fengshui* (usually translated as "geomancy" in English) axioms to choose locations of dwellings that highlighted the harmony between people and nature. Literally meaning "wind and water," *fengshui* is a collective expression of several esoteric principles, including *buzhai* (divination and orientation of a house site), *kanyu* (observation of the law of the sky and the earth), and *dili* (earth truth or

DOI: 10.4324/9781003122180-2

topographic patterns), which present the benefits the site and place offer to people's wealth, happiness, health, and longevity (Knapp & Lo, 2005).

Medical geographers tried to decipher therapeutic landscapes and historic places that have enduring reputations for healing and explored the unique aspects comprising the healing sense of places (Gesler, 2003; Williams, 1999). In ancient Greece, the sanctuary of Epidaurus was one of the most important healing sites, where sick individuals received dream healing by Asclepius, the god of medicine. A combination of environmental factors contributed to the healing reputation of Asclepian sanctuaries, including the pleasing solitariness of the site within untouched nature, fresh mountain air, supplies of spring water that symbolized purification, sacred building forms with long colonnade spaces, and spaces for socialization and leisure in nature (Gesler, 2003; Thompson & Goldin, 1975).

Water has traditionally been seen as being endowed with healing qualities. In Islamic culture, water has long been believed to be cooling, purifying, and solidifying the spiritual harmony of one's primordial status; indeed, the flowing rills of water and fountains are the most featured elements in Islamic gardens (Clark, 2004). Foley (2016) explored the roles of healing waters and spas as therapeutic landscapes in historic and contemporary Ireland. The term *spa* was actually invented by the Romans as an abbreviated version of the phrase *sanitas per acqua* or "health from water" (Jackson, 1990). The town of Spa (Belgium) and the mineral springs of Bath (UK) are historic places renowned for the therapeutic effects of their mineral-rich thermal waters. Thermal waters were believed to provide cures by soothing tired muscles, restoring balances among internal fluids, reducing pains, and softening the body's surfaces so that they can assimilate nutrients from food (Gesler, 2003; Jackson, 1990). The Roman baths were also important social centers of communities, combining various civic functions of hygienic care, church service, social interaction, and wellness in a single location (Verderber, 2010).

Trees, Flowers, and Herbs

Trees have been associated with many religious and spiritual qualities in different cultures due to their longevity, historical status, and continuity from one season to another (Squire, 2002). Trees, such as the oak and thorn, are viewed as connectors between people and the physical world to the God and spiritual world (Schroeder, 1991; Squire, 2002). Gautama Buddha attained enlightenment under the Bodhi tree at Bodh Gaya in India, and his teaching and meditation activities also took place in the forest; consequently, the Bodhi tree became a symbol of awakening, enlightenment, a status of ultimate mental tranquility, and the direct link to Buddhist mission (Nugteren, 2005). Certain flowers were also believed to have curing powers in ancient times. In many Asian cultures, the lotus is sacred, and its blossom means purity and achievement from suffering; meanwhile, in ancient

Egyptian culture, the lotus symbolized the sun and light, life, immortality, and resurrection (Ward, 1952).

Many cultures have also long employed plants to cure illnesses. The book *Compendium of Materia Medica* written by Shizhen Li (1518–1593) documented 1,892 plants, minerals, and other living organisms believed to have medicinal properties from the perspective of Chinese traditional medicine (Yaniv & Bachrach, 2005). Traditional indigenous medicine also adheres to the law of nature and employs herbs and diets to prevent and treat illness (Cohen, 2006). In the Middle Ages, herbs, flowers, and perfumes played a major role in daily life and were inextricably linked with magic and medicine (Hajar, 2012). The production of medicines during this era involved processing and distilling herbs at cloisters where pilgrims and sick people receive treatments or palliative care (Thompson & Goldin, 1975). Trees and herbs were planted in the cloister's *hortus conclusus*, a closed off/enclosed garden or orchard, to offer relief and treatments (Cooper Marcus & Barnes, 1999). In addition, headaches and aching joints were treated with fragrant plants, such as rose, lavender, sage, and hay (Hajar, 2012). The restorative values of such infirmary gardens can be found in the writing by abbot St. Bernard (1090–1153) for the monastery at Clairvaux:

> Within this enclosure, many and various trees, prolific with every sort of fruit, make a veritable grove, which lying next to the cells of those who are ill, lightens with no little solace to the infirmities of the brethren, while it offers to those who are strolling about a spacious walk, and to those overcome with the heat, a sweet place for repose .... The sick man sits upon the green lawn ... he is secure, shaded from the heat of the day. For the comfort of his pain all kinds of grass are fragrant in his nostrils. The lovely green of herb and tree nourishes his eyes ... the choir of painted birds caresses his ears ... the earth breathes with fruitfulness, and the invalid himself with eyes, ears, and nostrils, drinks in the delights of colors, songs and perfumes. (Comito, 1978, p. 177)

Salubrious Urban Landscape in the 19th Century

In the late 18th century, conditions in cities became crowded, polluted, and unhealthy. A wave of investigations into environmental issues in relation to public health emerged in Western societies around this time and became a prevailing civic topic in the 19th century (Davis, 1795). Miasmatic theory influenced the seeking of *salubrity*, which led to the urban open-air movement that included the legislation for urban parks and open-air walkways in English cities (Walker & Duffield, 1983). Medical topographies further identified the crucial link between environments and public health, such as the building styles, cleanliness of streets, paving conditions, flow of air, and the drainage systems of the city (Szczygiel &

Hewitt, 2000). The condition of cities was subsequently closely analyzed and mapped with the assistance of medical topography methods, which revealed a higher mortality rate in crowded city areas than rural areas, where nature was more accessible.

In America, since the mid-19th century, the pioneering landscape architects and medical professionals started to collaborate and seek sanitary reforms in urban environments (Martensen, 2009; Szczygiel & Hewitt, 2000). John Henry Rauch (1828–1894), a physician and environmental health officer in Chicago, conducted mortality statistics and environmental analyses that initiated the rural cemetery movement and ultimately affected the city's form (Szczygiel & Hewitt, 2000). Frederick Law Olmsted (1822–1903), known as the father of American landscape architecture, established urban park systems for many cities in the New England area and across the nation (Stevenson, 1977). Olmsted's prescient vision about preserving green and open spaces and connecting city inhabitants with nature may have stemmed from his earlier leadership for the US Sanitary Commission. Two main themes inspired Olmsted's work on salubrious urban landscape design: "his conviction that nature has healing and restorative psychological effects on the individual and his equally strong belief that nature is a civilizing force in society" (Nicholson, 2004, p. 337). Olmsted also tentatively established nature's therapeutic effects on mental health, fatigue restoration, and the maintenance of emotional and psychological well-being:

> The enjoyment of scenery employs the mind without fatigue and yet exercises it, tranquilizes it and yet enlivens it; and thus, through the influence of the mind over the body, gives the effect of refreshing rest and reinvigoration of the whole system. (Olmsted, 1865, as cited in Rybczynski, 1999, p. 258)

Nature's Healing Mechanism: Contemporary Studies and Schools of Thoughts

Therapeutic Landscapes through the Lens of Medical Geography

When explaining nature's healing effects, a significant amount of research comes from medical geography, a discipline of geography that investigates human–environmental relationships involving disease, nutrition, and healthcare systems (Earickson, 2009). The concept of "therapeutic landscapes" was first introduced by medical geographers to describe places, situations, locales, and milieus that "encompass both the physical and psychological environments associated with treatment or healing" (Williams, 1998, p. 1193). Such landscapes are reputed to have an "enduring reputation for achieving physical, mental and spiritual healing" (Gesler, 1993, p. 171). Places widely cited as therapeutic landscapes include Epidaurus in ancient Greece, Bath in England, Hot Springs in South Dakota, the village of Lourdes in France,

Denali National Park in Alaska, and New Zealand beaches, just to name a few (Geores, 1998; Gesler, 1996, 1998; Palka, 1999).

Based on a conceptual framework of humanism, the healing sense of place was centered in medical geography, and the achievement of the holistic healing sense of place occurs through the experience in several intertwining environments—namely, the natural environment, built environment, symbolic environment, and social environment (Gesler, 2003). Gesler (2003, p. 8) summarized aspects of the healing environments as follows:

- *Natural.* Aspects of the *natural* healing environment include belief in nature as healing, beauty, esthetic pleasure, remoteness, immersion in nature, and specific elements of nature.
- *Built.* Aspects of the *built* healing environment include sense of trust and security, affecting the senses, pride in building history, and symbolic power of design.
- *Symbolic.* Aspects of the *symbolic* healing environment include the creation of meaning, physical objects as symbols, and the importance of rituals.
- *Social.* Aspects of the *social* healing environment include equality in social relations, legitimization and marginalization, therapeutic community concept, and social support.

Evolutionary Perspectives

As early as the late 1960s, psychologists developed an interest in studying perception and environmental esthetics and raised questions about how people process a scene and whether natural features are more preferred than manmade materials in visual perception (Knecht, 2004). At least three prominent evolutionary perspectives emerged in this field: the habitat theory and the derived branches such as the prospect-refuge theory (Appleton, 1975; Orians, 1980, 1986; Orians & Heerwagen, 1992), the functionalist-evolutionary model (Kaplan, 1972, 1973; Kaplan & Kaplan, 1989), and the psychoevolutionary model (Ulrich, 1977, 1983); the latter two models rooted in environmental psychology and directly addressed nature restoration hypotheses (Parsons, 1991). Closely associated with visual esthetics and preferences, nature's therapeutic effects and the underlying mechanisms of restoration became a systematic investigation since 1970s. Three main schools of thoughts were coined to explain how and why nature can heal based primarily on evolutionary perspectives, as discussed in the following sections.

Biophilia and Biophilic Design

People adhered to the hunting-and-gathering model for the longest time prior to the invention of agriculture, accounting for more than 90% of human development history (Lee et al., 1999). The habitat theory and related prospect-refuge hypothesis (Appleton, 1975; Orians, 1980) claim that, through evolution, humans developed the ability to assess the environment for the selection of habitats that would ensure both vista (prospect) and protection (refuge) for hunting, sheltering, and survival. "Tropical savannahs, particularly those with irregular relief providing cliffs and caves, should have been the optimal environment for early man" (Orians, 1980, p. 57). A growing number of studies have found that people with diverse cultural backgrounds favor the savanna-like natural environments, which supports the hypothesis that humans possess an evolutionary adaption to life on the savanna of East Africa (Falk & Balling, 2010; Hagerhall et al., 2004). Thus, strong positive responses to, and the associated deeper benefits of, the savannah-like environment should have been selected in the evolution of human habitat choice mechanisms.

Habitat theories have been supported through several lines of indirect evidence, including historical accounts of landscape preferences, common practice in the choice and arrangement of esthetic vegetation, landscape painting, and environmental evaluation research (Hartig & Evans, 1993; Orians, 1980, 1986). Direct support to habitat theories have emerged from recent studies. For instance, Vincent and colleagues (2010) found that the prospect-refuge nature scenes are more effective than hazard nature scenes on pain relief and mood status among the simulated patients.

Habitat theories are inseparable in the discussion of biophilia. Wilson (1993, p. 31) defined biophilia as the "innately emotional affiliation of human beings to other living organisms." The biophilia hypothesis proclaims a human dependence on nature that "extends far beyond the simple issues of material and physical sustenance to encompass as well the human craving for aesthetic, intellectual, cognitive, and spiritual meaning and satisfaction" (Kellert, 1993, p. 20). According to the biophilic hypothesis, humans have developed a predisposition to pay attention and respond positively to certain natural content, such as food, vegetation, and water, as well as to configurations of settings that are favorable to survival or ongoing well-being during evolution (Ulrich et al., 1991). Roger Ulrich (1993) suggested that the rewards or advantages acquired in early human habitats led to positive/ approach (*biophilic*) responses while the dangers associated with natural creatures were sufficiently learned and adapted as fear-related/avoidance (*biophobic*) responses; both phobias have been supported through empirical evidence.

Concerning the physical environments, biophilia explains the foundational and universal need of contacting nature for people's health and well-being, which sets the ground for a series of important topics of varied scales and emphases, ranging from the values of connection to everyday nature to the preservation of the vastness of nature, resources and biodiversity, environmental ethics, social justice, inclusiveness and universal access to nature, and sustainable design and development that go beyond the low-environmental impact objectives (Heerwagen, 2009; Kellert, 2008).

Kellert et al. (2008) suggested using biophilic design principles to design restorative environments that support human health. Two core dimensions of biophilic design include organic or naturalistic forms and place-based or vernacular design; the former evokes one's innate preference to the universal beauty in nature and the latter reinforces the attachment to certain places due to comfort, familiarity, and domestic feelings. These two dimensions can be related to over 70 attributes of biophilic design that fall into six categories of elements, namely environmental features, natural shapes and forms, natural patterns and processes, light and space, place-based relationships, and the evolved human-nature relationships, as outlined in Kellert and colleagues' seminal edition *Biophilic Design* (2008, pp. 5–15).

Attention-Restoration Theory

In terms of a deeper explanation of nature's healing mechanism, Stephen Kaplan (1972, 1973) focused on the cognitive assessment of environments. To ensure humans' long-term survival, they had to become a highly visual animal capable of processing large quantities of visual landscape information. Through the course of evolution, humans adapted strong biases that preset contemporary humans' visual preferences and perceptions. Landscape scenes are generally preferred if they have attributes that are identifiable and legible and facilitate humans' comprehension of existing information. Another determinant of visual landscape preference is curiosity or exploration, which is consistent with the prerequisite that any living organism (both humans and animals) would have, such as acquiring landscape information and exploring the environment if it were to survive (Parsons, 1991; Ulrich, 1977).

The Kaplanesque school initially explored the psychological benefits of a wilderness experience, then further established the attention-restoration theory to explain nature's restorative effects on mental fatigue (Kaplan, 1984; Kaplan, 1992; Kaplan & Kaplan, 1989; Kaplan & Talbot, 1983). According to the theory, people process their surrounding information through two types of attention: directed attention and fascination or involuntary attention. Directed attention is employed in problem-solving and other mentally demanding tasks. Mental fatigue occurs when the capacity of directed attention is depleted, showing temporary symptoms of the brain malfunctioning that make people feel distracted, impatient, forgetful, or irritable, thereby resulting in a decline of working efficiency. Getting away from the attention-demanding tasks and using effortless and involuntary attention (fascination) instead could restore the mental capacity and recover from attentional fatigue (Kaplan, 1992; Kaplan & Berman, 2010; Kaplan & Kaplan, 1989). A natural environment, in providing high levels of restorative factors—namely, being away, extent, fascination, and compatibility—makes it an optimal restorative environment for mental fatigue recovery and human functioning (S. Kaplan, 1992; R. Kaplan, 1993, 2001;

Kaplan & Kaplan, 1989). People may get readily fascinated by natural features and in particular are thought to have an evolutionary basis; it would have been adaptive in a biological sense for humans to have their attention effortlessly captured by environmental features relevant for survival (Hartig et al., 2008).

The four restorative factors as provided by nature were clearly explained by Kaplan (1992, pp. 137–138; 1995, p. 173) as follows:

- *Being Away.* Being in some other setting makes it more likely that one can think of other things. People often talk of having to get away or needing a change when they are exasperated by the accumulation of mental fatigue.
- *Extent.* Restorative settings are often described as being "in a whole different world." The environment must be rich enough and coherent enough so that it constitutes a whole other world. Two properties are important to this experience: connectedness and scope. Scope requires that the environment be experienced as large enough that one can move around in it. To have connectedness, the various parts of the environment must be perceived as belonging to a larger whole.
- *Fascination.* In addition to the need for extent, restorative experiences depend upon interest or fascination. A fascinating stimulus is one that calls forth involuntary attention that allows one to function without using directed attention.
- *Compatibility.* The final component of the restorative concept calls upon the compatibility among the environmental patterns, the individual's inclinations, and the actions required by the environment. In a compatible environment, what one wants to do and is inclined to do are what is needed in and supported by the environment. When what intuitively feels right is what the situation requires, one's relationship to the environment takes on an effortless quality that can be deeply restorative.

Extensive research has discussed the attention-restoration theory by exploring the nature's restorative qualities in the wilderness as well as a much wider range of urban conditions, from public open spaces and urban parklands to nearby nature in the school, workplace, and residential contexts. Hartig and colleagues (1997) developed the Perceived Restorativeness Scale (PRS) to measure nature's restorative effects based on the attention-restoration theory. This tool has been validated by many studies (Herzog et al., 2003; Ivarsson & Hagerhall, 2008). Generally speaking, natural settings—whether wildness or urban parks—provide better restorative qualities than hardscapes (Berto, 2005; Herzog et al., 2003; Laumann et al., 2001). The amount or density of trees is a positive predictor of people's esthetic preferences (Jiang et al., 2015; Kaplan, 2007; Wang et al., 2019). However, some research findings expanded the scope of the *extent* attribute and found that the restorative quality of urban greenspaces does not depend exclusively on size. Well-designed pocket parks in dense cities may also have high restorative value ratings if they are greener or composed of a larger ratio of planting materials (Nordh et al., 2009). In addition, the presence of water or flowers tends to significantly predict a setting's restorative potential (Gao et al., 2019; Voelker & Kistemann, 2013; Wang et al., 2019).

Stress Reduction and the Esthetic-Affective Model

Ulrich (1979) reiterated Olmsted's (1870, p. 23) belief that nature in urban environments brings "tranquility and rest to the mind," but the "nature tranquility hypothesis" should be rigorously tested and evaluated (p. 17). A then-novel experiment was conducted by dividing 46 participants with mentally stressed status into two groups to watch a slide presentation of either nature scenes dominated by green vegetation or urban scenes lacking nature elements (Ulrich, 1979). Participants' level of emotional and anxiety scores was measured before and after the slide presentation and revealed that exposure to urban views had more aggravating than mitigating effects than nature scenes (Ulrich, 1979).

Although Ulrich (1983) also posited the Kaplans' cognitive assessment of environmental information, his *psychoevolutionary* model, also referred as the esthetic-affective model or stress-reduction theory (Abkar et al., 2010; Jiang et al., 2020; Kaufman, 2018), emphasizes the affective responses to the visual perception of an environment. Affective response is defined as the like–dislike emotion in association with pleasurable feelings and physiological responses elicited by the visual encounter with a natural setting, which could be independent of and prior to cognition (Ulrich, 1983; Zajonc, 1980). Affects are innate, cross-cultural adaptions composed of facial, experiential, cognitive, and neurophysiological components (Ulrich, 1983). Certain broad classes of natural features, such as water and vegetation, can produce visual ambiances that quickly elicit affective reactions prior to processing the visual information using cognition. The initial affect reaction then promotes a reduction in sympathetic nervous system arousal and serves as an action impulse for behaviors or functioning that foster well-being, thereby reducing stress (Kaufman, 2018; Ulrich, 1983).

Esthetic preference is interpreted as affect within the broad pleasantness dimension of emotion; esthetic affect could be a response to elements having either real or symbolic significance for survival as presented in many nature views (Appleton, 1975; Ulrich, 1983). As asserted by Donald Ruggles (2017, p. 13), "we (humans) respond to a broad and dramatic view as beautiful and inspiring as a result of 2.4 million years of evolution. We feel intuitively that it is safe, bountiful and full of pleasure."

Several visual properties influence the esthetic preference and affective responses to the environment, including complexity, structural properties, focality, depth, ground surface texture, threat/tension, deflected vistas, and water as strong features that elicit the liking affect. Specifically, natural scenes with the following visual properties should be preferred (Ulrich, 1983, p. 105):

- Complexity is moderate to high.
- The complexity has structural properties that establish a focal point, and other order or patterning is present.
- There is a moderate to high level of depth that can be perceived unambiguously.
- The ground surface texture tends to be homogenous and even and is appraised as conducive to movement.
- A deflected vista is present, suggesting the possibility of further discovery.
- Appraised threat is negligible or absent.
- A water feature is present.

Stress in Ulrich's (1999) model is used "in a broad sense to refer to a process of responding to events and environmental features that are challenging, demanding, or threatening to well-being. The demanding events and environmental features are called stressors" (p. 32). Environmental stressors may include crowding and noise in the urban context (Evans & Cohen, 1987), while stressors in the hospital environment include unknown diagnostic procedures, pain, loss of control or privacy, noise, wayfinding challenges in the highly institutional environment, and so on. Anxiety and stress can cause people's attention and performance to decline, thereby leading to psychological/emotional, physiological, neuroendocrine, and behavioral changes (Ulrich, 1999). The stress-reducing effects of the visual encounter with nature take place in such esthetic-affective procedures as matter-of-unconscious processes and affect the emotion-driven parts of the brain that inform people when to relax (Grahn et al., 2010; Ulrich, 1979, 1999). For individuals experiencing stress or anxiety, most unthreatening natural views may be more arousal reducing and tend to elicit more positively toned emotional reactions, thereby being more restorative in a psychophysiological sense (Ulrich, 1983). Rooted in the stress-reduction theory, Ulrich has made seminal contributions in healthcare environmental design, which will be discussed later in the book.

Toward an Integrative Framework

As Hartig and colleagues (1993, 2008) discussed, nature restoration theories under the biophilic umbrella have been dominated by two main positions: one emphasizing physiological stress reduction (Ulrich, 1984; Ulrich et al., 1991) and the other concerning the recovery of attentional fatigue (Kaplan & Kaplan, 1989). Parsons (1991) has compared the similarities and differences of the Kaplanesque and Ulrichean models and identified the primary differences between the two. Ulrich proposed that the initial response to an environment is one of generalized affect, which can be independent of and primary to cognition, emphasizing that attentional decline is a consequence of stress. In contrast, the Kaplanesque model assumes that people's preference to natural environments relies heavily on the cognitive processes; nature has restorative effects because it supports the information people need and provides relief from mental fatigue (Kaplan, 1995).

Despite some differences, the two schools of thoughts overlap and share some foundational propositions. Both schools emphasize that the esthetic qualities of nature scenes play an indispensable role in restoration and stress reduction. People's visual preference for, and affective response to, nature environments warrant its therapeutic benefits (Gao et al., 2019). As research has demonstrated, a strong positive relationship exists between people's esthetic preference for an environment and the environment's restorative potential (Herzog et al., 2003; Jiang, 2015; Van den Berg et al., 2003; Wang et al., 2019). However, it was not clear whether the restorative benefits result from exposure to nature stimuli per se or result from viewing a beautiful, highly preferred stimulus, until recent studies found a preference-based account of affective benefits. Nature offers a positive effect on the affect state only because it is beautiful and, thus, highly preferred. If a nature scene was sufficiently low on esthetics or compared to an equally preferred urban scene, it would fail to sustain additional benefits of nature on the affective state (Meidenbauer et al., 2020). According to the latest findings, even nature with very high esthetics did not elicit larger affective responses than other equally preferred stimuli, suggesting there was not an additional benefit to the affective state of viewing natural scenery per se (Meidenbauer et al., 2020).

Hartig and Evans (1993) and Kaplan (1995) proposed a logical integration of the stress-reduction and attention-restoration theories, which placed both directed attention and stress in the larger context of the human–environment relationship. The examination of the factors leading to stress—namely, harm and resource inadequacy—indicated that cognition and rapid, unconscious information processing play a role when a stress response occurs. The decline of directed attention as a resource inadequacy can lead to stress. In fact, under a wide range of circumstances, the resource deficiencies and stress responses frequently occur together, and "the frequent co-occurrence could readily lead to the assumption that one concept subsumes the other" (Kaplan, 1995, p. 178). The integrated framework explains many of the seemly conflicting scenarios. For instance, it explains how one can enjoy what one is doing, be good at it, and confident of a positive outcome but still be exhausted from it; it also explains how the same task can be stressful at one time and not at another—an individual already fatigued (experiencing resource inadequacy) could find a task stressful even though the same individual in a rested state might consider the same tasks to be manageable (Kaplan, 1995).

Nature Restoration: New Perspectives and New Tools

Along with the consistent research efforts on the topics of nature resto-ration, new research tools and new perspectives have emerged in recent years. Both schools have been traditionally associated with the visual attributes of the environment; however, the multi-sensory stimuli provided by nature, including haptic, auditory and olfactory elements, could also play important roles in restoration and stress reduction (Cohen, 2009). Researchers have postulated that a common preference exists for natural sounds, and recent studies have found that the sounds of nature can pro-mote the restoration of attention—most notably in response to birdsong (Alvarsson et al., 2010; Medvedev et al., 2015; Pilcher et al., 2009; Ratcliffe et al., 2013, 2016). Odorant stimuli from nature, such as methyl salicy-late (wintergreen scent), have been universally rated as smelling healthful (Dalton, 1996, 1999).

Recent studies have further expanded the knowledge boundary and depth of nature restoration. Beyond relieving from mental fatigue and acute stress, a wide range of health outcomes have been proven as a result of varying forms of nature exposure among different populations, thereby expanding the research arena of nature restoration to public health and preventive healthcare. More and more health benefits of nature have been supported through empirical studies, including improved air quality, asthma, and atopic sensitization (Eisenman et al., 2019; Lambert et al., 2018), cardiovascular health (Yeager et al., 2020), dementia and neuro-logical health (Lakhani et al., 2019; Mmako et al., 2020), birth outcomes (Akaraci et al., 2020), mortality rate (Rojas-Rueda et al., 2019), sleep qual-ity (Shin et al., 2020), obesity prevention and the maintenance of a healthy body mass index level (Ghimire et al., 2017; Lachowycz & Jones, 2011; Luo et al., 2020), and nature's impacts on the mental health and well-being for children, adolescents, adults, the elderly, and marginalized populations (Akpınar, 2019; Houlden et al., 2018; Vanaken & Danckaerts, 2018).

Three forms of nature exposure have been found to be beneficial to peo-ple's health status according to the levels of person–nature engagement; these three forms are (1) passive engagement: visual contact with nature through a window or seeing a nature-themed painting/artwork; (2) inciden-tal presence: simply being present in nearby nature or a convenient nat-ural setting, such as an interior planting installation or a courtyard; and (3) active participation and involvement with nature, such as gardening and physical exercises in a natural environment, also known as green exer-cise (Abkar et al., 2010; Pretty, 2004; Pretty et al., 2005; Ward-Thompson, 2011). Based on Pretty's (2004) framework, a list of health benefits/outcomes of nature has been compiled regarding different levels of people–nature engagement. It is more of an outline than an explicit list that demonstrates a broad spectrum of people–nature relationships, as shown in Figure 2.1. More in-depth synthetizations of nature's health benefits can be found in

Passive Engagement

Visual Contact with Nature

Windows at home
- Enhanced residential satisfaction (Kaplan, 2001)
- Improved satisfaction and well-being (Kaplan, 2001)
- Green views from home can facilitate children's cognitive functioning and their capacity of thinking (Taylor et al., 2002)

Windows at workplace
- Enhanced staff satisfaction (Leather et al., 1998)
- People having window seats show fewer illness, be less frustrated, more patient and enthusiastic about work (Pretty, 2004)
- Better job performance (Lottrup et al., 2013)

Windows in the healthcare environment
- Shorter length of stay and fewer pain reliever (Ulrich, 1984)
- Higher satisfaction during hospitalization (Verderber, 1986)
- Higher level of alertness for nurses (Pati et al., 2008)
- Enhanced mood, reduced stress (Jiang et al., 2017)
- Reduced pain and enhanced mood status (Vincent et al., 2010)

Nature painting/art in the healthcare environment
- Positive distraction and preference (Ulrich, 1999)
- Calming behaviors (Lankston et al., 2010)

Incidental Presence

Being in the Presence of Nearby Nature

Interior plants in the healthcare environment
- Reduced patient stress (Baldwin, 2012)
- Reduced physical discomfort (Lohr & Pearson-Mims, 2000)

Roadside vegetation
- Reduced stress and mood enhancement (Parsons, et al., 1998)
- Improved mental stauts and restoration for drivers (Jiang et al., 2020)

Nearby nature in residential areas
- Improved health status and well-being (Stigsdotter et al., 2010)
- Lower likelihood of obesity, lower stress (Nielsen & Hansen, 2007)
- Higher perceived sense of safety (Kuo et al., 1998)

Interior plants/gardens/courtyards at workplace
- Better job performance (Raanaas et al., 2011)
- Stress reduction (Stigsdotter & Grahn, 2004)
- Improved job satisfaction (Dravigne et al., 2008)

Healing gardens in the healthcare environment
- Stress reduction and mood change (Cooper Marcus & Sachs, 2013)
- Enhanced rehabilitation progress (Adevi et al., 2018)
- Enhanced satisfaction (Whitehouse et al., 2001)

Active Participation

Horticulture therapy gardening/activities
- Enhanced living quality for the elderly (Detweiler et al., 2012)
- Stress reduction (Eriksson et al., 2011)
- Occupational therapy for patients with dementia (Chaplin, 2003)

Gardening and Green Exercise

Green exercises
- Healthy weight status/BMI (Akpinar, 2019)
- Improved physical and mental health; improved self-esteem and mood (Barton & Pretty, 2010; Pretty et al., 2005)

HEALTH BENEFITS/ OUTCOMES

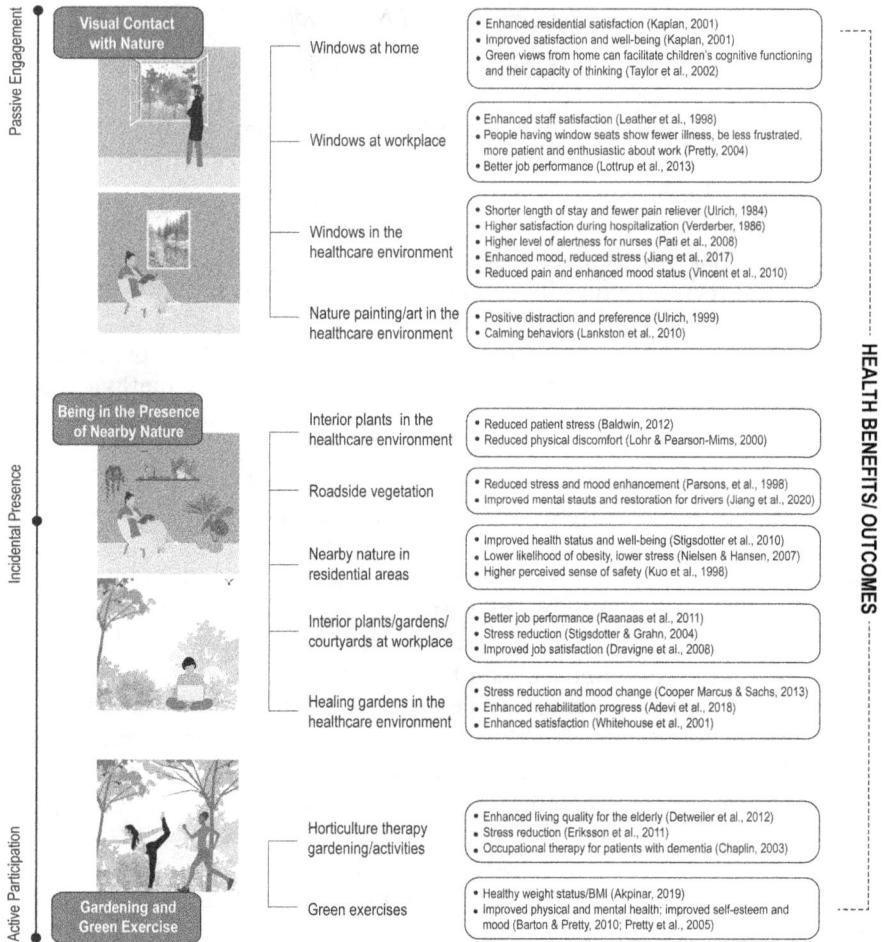

The theoretical framework of this diagram was adapted from Pretty's (2004, p. 68) three levels of engagement with nature. The first is viewing nature as through a window or in a painting. The second is being in the presence of usually nearby nature, which is incidental to some other activity, such as reading on a garden seat. The third is active participation and involvement with nature, such as gardening or running in nature.

Figure 2.1 Levels of people–nature engagement and the associated health benefits/ outcomes

Source: Drawn by Shan Jiang and Udday Datta

many meta-analyses and systematic reviews (Hartig et al., 2014; Soga et al., 2017; Twohig-Bennett & Jones, 2018).

Technology, methods, and tools have also been greatly advanced in the recent decade, which has facilitated waves of new findings around the topics of nature restoration. In the human scale, the effects of viewing nature have been examined by a series of physiological indicators, such as the participant's heart period, muscle tension, skin conductance and pulse transit time (Ulrich et al., 1991); blood pressure (Jiang, 2015; Vincent et al., 2010); electromyography (EMG), electroencephalography (EEG), and blood volume pulse (BVP) (Chang & Chen, 2005); salivary cortisol (Roe et al., 2013; Thompson et al., 2012); and serum hydroperoxide levels (Sugaya et al., 2011). Immersive virtual environment (IVE) techniques offer fully immersive, simulated nature environments and supplement the traditional lab experiments using imagery simulations (Browning et al., 2020; Joseph et al., 2020). Using magnetic resonance imaging (MRI), Dadvand et al. (2018) identified the association between greenspace exposure and brain development and functioning; meanwhile, other researchers have utilized eye-tracking techniques to further reveal the mechanisms in attention distraction and restoration (Conniff & Craig, 2016; Stevenson et al., 2019). In the spatio-temporal approach, the geographic information system (GIS) and remote sensing techniques revealed the dynamics between population health and the proximity of green outdoor spaces (De Vries et al., 2003; McCracken et al., 2016; Su et al., 2019). Data-mining techniques have also been utilized to establish models to predict urban park esthetics and their mental restoration potential (Jahani & Saffariha, 2020).

References

Abkar, M., Kamal, M., Maulan, S., & Mariapan, M. (2010). Influences of viewing nature through windows. *Australian Journal of Basic and Applied Sciences*, *4*(10), 5346–5351.

Adevi, A. A., Uvnäs-Moberg, K., & Grahn, P. (2018). Therapeutic interventions in a rehabilitation garden may induce temporary extrovert and/or introvert behavioural changes in patients, suffering from stress-related disorders. *Urban Forestry & Urban Greening*, *30*, 182–193.

Akaraci, S., Feng, X., Suesse, T., Jalaludin, B., & Astell-Burt, T. (2020). A systematic review and meta-analysis of associations between green and blue spaces and birth outcomes. *International Journal of Environmental Research and Public Health*, *17*(8), 2949.

Akpınar, A. (2019). Green exercise: How are characteristics of urban green spaces associated with adolescents' physical activity and health? *International Journal of Environmental Research and Public Health*, *16*(21), 4281.

Alvarsson, J. J., Wiens, S., & Nilsson, M. E. (2010). Stress recovery during exposure to nature sound and environmental noise. *International Journal of Environmental Research and Public Health*, *7*(3), 1036–1046.

Appleton, J. (1975). *The experience of landscape*. Wiley.

Baldwin, A. L. (2012). How do plants in hospital waiting rooms reduce patient stress? *The Journal of Alternative and Complementary Medicine*, *18*(4), 1–2. 10.1089/acm.2012.0116

Barton, J., & Pretty, J. (2010). What is the best dose of nature and green exercise for improving mental health? A multi-study analysis. *Environmental Science & Technology*, *44*(10), 3947–3955.

Berto, R. (2005). Exposure to restorative environments helps restore attentional capacity. *Journal of Environmental Psychology*, *25*(3), 249–259.

Browning, M. H., Saeidi-Rizi, F., McAnirlin, O., Yoon, H., & Pei, Y. (2020). *The role of methodological choices in the effects of experimental exposure to simulated natural landscapes on human health and cognitive performance: A systematic review. Environment and Behavior*, https://journals.sagepub.com/doi/abs/10.1177/0013916520906481

Chang, C. Y., & Chen, P. K. (2005). Human response to window views and indoor plants in the workplace. *HortScience, 40*(5), 1354–1359.

Chaplin, R. (2003). Occupational therapy interventions. In R. C. Baldwin, & M. Murray (Eds.), *Younger people with dementia: A multidisciplinary approach* (pp. 74–85). CRC Press.

Clark, E. (2004). *The art of the Islamic garden.* The Crowood Press.

Cohen, K. (2006). *Honoring the medicine: An essential guide to Native American healing.* Ballantine Books.

Cohen, R. (2009). *The science of healing with Dr. Esther Sternberg [Film].* Produced by Matt and Renard Cohen: Movies & TV.

Cooper Marcus, C., & Sachs, N. A. (2013). *Therapeutic landscapes: An evidence-based approach to designing healing gardens and restorative outdoor spaces.* John Wiley & Sons.

Comito, T. (1978). *The idea of the garden in the renaissance.* Rutgers University Press.

Conniff, A., & Craig, T. (2016). A methodological approach to understanding the wellbeing and restorative benefits associated with greenspace. *Urban Forestry & Urban Greening, 19*, 103–109.

Dadvand, P., Pujol, J., Macià, D., Martínez-Vilavella, G., Blanco-Hinojo, L., Mortamais, M., Alvarez-Pedrerol, M., Fenoll, R., Esnaola, M., Dalmai-Bueno, A., Lopez-Vicente, M., Basagana, X., Jerrett, M., Nieuwenhuijsen, M. J., & Sunyer, J. (2018). The association between lifelong greenspace exposure and 3-dimensional brain magnetic resonance imaging in Barcelona schoolchildren. *Environmental Health Perspectives, 126*(2), 027012.

Dalton, P. (1996). Odor perception and beliefs about risk. *Chemical Senses, 21*(4), 447–458.

Dalton, P. (1999). Cognitive influences on health symptoms from acute chemical exposure. *Health Psychology, 18*(6), 579–590.

Davis, M. L. (1795). *A brief account of the epidemical fever which lately prevailed in the city of New York: With the different proclamations, reports and letters of Gov. Jay, Gov. Mifflin, the Health Committee of New York, &c. upon the subject: to which is added, an accurate list of the names of those who have died of the disease, from July 29, to Nov. 1.* Matthew L. Davis, no. 151 Water Street.

De Vries, S., Verheij, R. A., Groenewegen, P. P., & Spreeuwenberg, P. (2003). Natural environments—Healthy environments? An exploratory analysis of the relationship between greenspace and health. *Environment and Planning A, 35*(10), 1717–1731.

Detweiler, M. B., Sharma, T., Detweiler, J. G., Murphy, P. F., Lane, S., Carman, J., Chudhary, A. S., Halling, M. H., & Kim, K. Y. (2012). What is the evidence to support the use of therapeutic gardens for the elderly? *Psychiatry Investigation, 9*(2), 100.

Earickson, R. (2009) Medical geography. In R. Kitchin, & N. Thrift (Eds.), *International encyclopedia of human geography* (Vol. 1; pp. 9–20). Elsevier.

Eisenman, T. S., Churkina, G., Jariwala, S. P., Kumar, P., Lovasi, G. S., Pataki, D. E., Weinberger, K. R., & Whitlow, T. H. (2019). Urban trees, air quality, and asthma: An interdisciplinary review. *Landscape and Urban Planning, 187*, 47–59.

Eriksson, T., Westerberg, Y., & Jonsson, H. (2011). Experiences of women with stress-related ill health in a therapeutic gardening program. *Canadian Journal of Occupational Therapy, 78*(5), 273–281.

Evans, G. W., & Cohen, S. (1987). Environmental stress. In D. Stokols, & I. Altman (Eds.), *Handbook of environmental psychology* (pp. 571–610). John Wiley.

Falk, J. H., & Balling, J. D. (2010). Evolutionary influence on human landscape preference. *Environment and Behavior, 42*(4), 479–493.

Foley, R. (2016). *Healing waters: Therapeutic landscapes in historic and contemporary Ireland.* Routledge.

Gao, T., Zhang, T., Zhu, L., Gao, Y., & Qiu, L. (2019). Exploring psychophysiological restoration and individual preference in the different environments based on virtual reality. *International Journal of Environmental Research and Public Health, 16*(17), 3102. http://dx.doi.org/10.3390/ijerph16173102

Gesler, W. M. (1993). Therapeutic landscapes: Theory and a case study of Epidauros, Greece. *Environment and Planning D: Society and Space, 11*(2), 171–189.

Gesler, W. M. (1996). Lourdes: Healing in a place of pilgrimage. *Health and Place, 2*, 95–105.

Gesler, W. M. (1998). Bath's reputation as a healing place. In R. Kearns, & W. Gesler (Eds.), *Putting health into place* (pp. 17–35). Syracuse University Press.

Gesler, W. M. (2003). *Healing places.* Rowman & Littlefield.

Geores, M.E. (1998). Surviving on metaphor: How 'Health Hot Springs' created and sustained a town. In R. Kearns and W. M. Gesler (Eds.). *Putting health into place: Landscape, identity and well-being.* Syracuse University Press, 36–52.

Ghimire, R., Ferreira, S., Green, G. T., Poudyal, N. C., Cordell, H. K., & Thapa, J. R. (2017). Green space and adult obesity in the United States. *Ecological Economics, 136*, 201–212.

Grahn, P., Ivarsson, C. T., Stigsdotter, U. K., & Bengtsson, I. L. (2010). In C. W. Thompson, P. Aspinall, & S. Bell (Eds.), *Innovative approaches to researching landscape and health: Open space: People space 2.* Routledge.

Hagerhall, C. M., Purcell, T., & Taylor, R. (2004). Fractal dimension of landscape silhouette outlines as a predictor of landscape preference. *Journal of Environmental Psychology, 24*(2), 247–255.

Hajar, R. (2012). The air of history (part II) medicine in the middle ages. *Heart Views, 13*(4), 158–162. 10.4103/1995-705X.105744

Hartig, T., & Evans, G. W. (1993). Psychological foundations of nature experience. In T. Garling, & R. G. Golledge (Eds.), *Behavior and environment: Psychological and geographical approaches* (pp. 427–457). Amsterdam: Elsevier/North Holland.

Hartig, T., Bringslimark, T., & Patil, G. G. (2008). Chapter 9: Restorative environmental design: What, when, where, and for whom? In S. R. Kellert, J. H. Jeerwagen, & M. L. Mador (Eds.), *Biophilic design: The theory, science, and practice of brining buildings to life* (pp. 133–151). Hoboken, NJ: John Wiley & Sons, Inc.

Hartig, T., Korpela, K., Evans, G. W., & Gärling, T. (1997). A measure of restorative quality in environments. *Scandinavian Housing and Planning Research, 14*(4), 175–194.

Hartig, T., Mitchell, R., De Vries, S., & Frumkin, H. (2014). Nature and health. *Annual Review of Public Health, 35*, 207–228.

Heerwagen, J. (2009). Biophilia, health, and well-being. In Campbell, L. & Wiesen, A. (Eds.). *Restorative commons: Creating health and well-being through urban landscapes.* USDA Forest Service Northern Research Station, pp. 38–57. Retrieved from https://www.fs.usda.gov/treesearch/pubs/18810

Herzog, T. R., Maguire, P., & Nebel, M. B. (2003). Assessing the restorative components of environments. *Journal of Environmental Psychology*, *23*(2), 159–170.

Hippocrates. (2010). *On airs, waters and places* (F. Adams, Trans.). Kessinger Publishing, LLC.

Houlden, V., Weich, S., Porto de Albuquerque, J., Jarvis, S., & Rees, K. (2018). The relationship between greenspace and the mental wellbeing of adults: A systematic review. *PLoS One*, *13*(9), e0203000.

Ivarsson, C. T., & Hagerhall, C. M. (2008). The perceived restorativeness of gardens–Assessing the restorativeness of a mixed built and natural scene type. *Urban Forestry & Urban Greening*, *7*(2), 107–118.

Jackson, R. (1990). Waters and spas in the classical world. In R. Porter (Ed.), *Medical history* (Supplement No. 10; pp. 1–13). Wellcome Institute for the History of Medicine.

Jahani, A., & Saffariha, M. (2020). Aesthetic preference and mental restoration prediction in urban parks: An application of environmental modeling approach. *Urban Forestry & Urban Greening*, *54*, 126775.

Jiang, B., He, J., Chen, J., Larsen, L., & Wang, H. (2020). Perceived green at speed: A simulated driving experiment raises new questions for attention restoration theory and stress reduction theory. *Environment and Behavior*. https://doi.org/ 10.1177/0013916520947111

Jiang, B., Larsen, L., Deal, B., & Sullivan, W. C. (2015). A dose–response curve describing the relationship between tree cover density and landscape preference. *Landscape and Urban Planning*, *139*, 16–25.

Jiang, S. (2015). Encouraging engagement with therapeutic landscapes: Using transparent spaces to optimize stress reduction in urban health facilities. *All Dissertations*. 1495. https://tigerprints.clemson.edu/all_dissertations/1495

Joseph, A., Browning, M. H. E. M., & Jiang, S. (2020). Using immersive virtual environments (IVEs) to conduct environmental design research: A primer and decision framework. *Health Environments Research & Design Journal*, *13*(3), 11–25. https://doi.org/10.1177/1937586720924787

Kaplan, R. (1984). Impact of urban nature: A theoretical analysis. *Urban Ecology*, *8*(3), 189–197.

Kaplan, R. (1993). The role of nature in the context of the workplace. *Landscape and Urban Planning*, *26*(1), 193–201.

Kaplan, R. (2001). The nature of the view from home psychological benefits. *Environment and Behavior*, *33*(4), 507–542.

Kaplan, R. (2007). Employees' reactions to nearby nature at their workplace: The wild and the tame. *Landscape and Urban Planning*, *82*(1–2), 17–24

Kaplan, R., & Kaplan, S. (1989). *The experience of nature: A psychological perspective*. CUP Archive.

Kaplan, S. (1972). The challenge of environmental psychology: A proposal for a new functionalism. *American Psychologist*, *27*(2), 140–143.

Kaplan, S. (1973). Cognitive maps, human needs, and the designed environment. In W. Preiser (Ed.), *Environmental design research* (pp. 275–283). Dowden, Hutchinson, and Ross.

Kaplan, S. (1992). The restorative environment: Nature and human experience. In *Role of horticulture in human well-being and social development: A national symposium* (pp. 134–142). Timber Press.

Kaplan, S. (1995). The restorative benefits of nature: Toward an integrative framework. *Journal of Environmental Psychology, 15*(3), 169–182.

Kaplan, S., & Berman, M. G. (2010). Directed attention as a common resource for executive functioning and self-regulation. *Perspectives on Psychological Science, 5*(1), 43–57.

Kaplan, S., & Talbot, J. F. (1983). Psychological benefits of a wilderness experience. In *Behavior and the natural environment* (pp. 163–203). Springer.

Kaufman, J. A. (2018). Nature, mind, and medicine: A model for mind–body healing. *Explore, 14*(4), 268–276.

Kellert, S. R., Jeerwagen, J. H., & Mador, M. L. (Eds.). (2008). *Biophilic design: The theory, science, and practice of brining buildings to life.* Hoboken, NJ: John Wiley & Sons, Inc.

Knapp, R. G., & Lo, K. Y. (Eds.). (2005). *House, home, family: Living and being Chinese.* University of Hawaii Press.

Knecht, C. (2004). Urban nature and well-being: Some empirical support and design implications. *Berkeley Planning Journal, 17*(1).

Kuo, F. E., Bacaicoa, M., & Sullivan, W. C. (1998). Transforming inner-city landscapes: Trees, sense of safety, and preference. *Environment and Behavior, 30*(1), 28–59.

Lachowycz, K., & Jones, A. P. (2011). Greenspace and obesity: A systematic review of the evidence. *Obesity Reviews, 12*(5), e183–e189.

Lakhani, A., Norwood, M., Watling, D. P., Zeeman, H., & Kendall, E. (2019). Using the natural environment to address the psychosocial impact of neurological disability: A systematic review. *Health & Place, 55*, 188–201.

Lambert, K. A., Bowatte, G., Tham, R., Lodge, C. J., Prendergast, L. A., Heinrich, J., Abramson, M. J., Dharmage, S. C., & Erbas, B. (2018). Greenspace and atopic sensitization in children and adolescents—a systematic review. *International Journal of Environmental Research and Public Health, 15*(11), 2539.

Lankston, L., Cusack, P., Fremantle, C., & Isles, C. (2010). Visual art in hospitals: Case studies and review of the evidence. *Journal of the Royal Society of Medicine, 103*(12), 490–499.

Laumann, K., Gärling, T., & Stormark, K. M. (2001). Rating scale measures of restorative components of environments. *Journal of Environmental Psychology, 21*(1), 31–44.

Lee, R. B., Daly, R. H., & Daly, R. (Eds.). (1999). *The Cambridge encyclopedia of hunters and gatherers.* Cambridge University Press.

Lohr, V. I., & Pearson-Mims, C. H. (2000). Physical discomfort may be reduced in the presence of interior plants. *HortTechnology, 10*(1), 53–58.

Lottrup, L., Grahn, P., & Stigsdotter, U. K. (2013). Workplace greenery and perceived level of stress: Benefits of access to a green outdoor environment at the workplace. *Landscape and Urban Planning, 110*, 5–11.

Luo, Y. N., Huang, W. Z., Liu, X. X., Markevych, I., Bloom, M. S., Zhao, T., Heinrich, J., Yang, B.-Y., & Dong, G. H. (2020). Greenspace with overweight and obesity: A systematic review and meta-analysis of epidemiological studies up to 2020. *Obesity Reviews, 21*(11), e13078.

Marcus, C. C., & Barnes, M. (Eds.). (1999). *Healing gardens: Therapeutic benefits and design recommendations.* John Wiley & Sons.

Martensen, R. (2009). Landscape designers, doctors, and the making of healthy urban spaces in 19th century America. In L. K. Campbell, & A. Wiesen (Eds.), *Restorative commons: Creating health and well-being through urban landscapes* (Vol. 39; pp. 26–37). USDA Forest Service.

McCracken, D. S., Allen, D. A., & Gow, A. J. (2016). Associations between urban greenspace and health-related quality of life in children. *Preventive Medicine Reports, 3*, 211–221.

Medvedev, O., Shepherd, D., & Hautus, M. J. (2015). The restorative potential of soundscapes: A physiological investigation. *Applied Acoustics, 96*, 20–26.

Meidenbauer, K. L., Stenfors, C. U. D., Bratman, G. N., Gross, J. J., Schertz, K. E., Choe, K. W., & Berman, M. G. (2020) The affective benefits of nature exposure: What's nature got to do with it? *Journal of Environmental Psychology, 72*, 101498. 10.1016/j.jenvp.2020.101498

Mmako, N. J., Courtney-Pratt, H., & Marsh, P. (2020). Green spaces, dementia and a meaningful life in the community: A mixed studies review. *Health & Place, 63*, 102344.

Nicholson, C. J. (2004). Elegance and grass roots: The neglected philosophy of Frederick Law Olmsted. *Transactions of the Charles S. Peirce Society, 40*(2), 335–348.

Nielsen, T. S., & Hansen, K. B. (2007). Do green areas affect health? Results from a Danish survey on the use of green areas and health indicators. *Health & Place, 13*(4), 839–850.

Nordh, H., Hartig, T., Hagerhall, C. M., & Fry, G. (2009). *Components of small urban parks that predict the possibility for restoration. Urban Forestry & Urban Greening, 8*(4), 225–235.

Nugteren, A. (2005). *Belief, bounty, and beauty: rituals around sacred trees in India.* Brill.

Olmsted, F. L. (1865). *The value and care of parks. Report to the Congress of the State of California.* [Reprinted in Nash, R. (Ed.). (1976). *The American environment* (pp. 18–24). Addison-Wesley.]

Olmsted, F. L. (1870). *Public parks and the enlargement of towns.* Riverside Press.

Orians, G. H. (1980). Habitat selection: General theory and applications to human behavior. In J. S. Lockard (Ed.), *The evolution of human social behavior* (pp. 49–66). Elsevier.

Orians, G. H. (1986). An ecological and evolutionary approach to landscape aesthetics. In E. C. Penning-Rowsell, & D. Lowenthal (Eds.), *Landscape meanings and values* (pp. 3–22). Allen & Unwin.

Orians, G. H., & Heerwagen, J. H. (1992). Evolved responses to landscapes. In J. H. Barkow, L. Cosmides, & J. Tooby (Eds.), *The adapted mind: Evolutionary psychology and the generation of culture* (pp. 555–579). Oxford University Press.

Palka, E. J. (1999). Accessible wilderness as a therapeutic landscape: Experiencing the nature of Denali National Park, Alaska. In A. Williams (Ed.), *Therapeutic landscapes: The dynamic between place and wellness* (pp. 29–51). University Press of America.

Parsons, R. (1991). The potential influences of environmental perception on human health. *Journal of Environmental Psychology, 11*(1), 1–23.

Parsons, R., Tassinary, L. G., Ulrich, R. S., Hebl, M. R., & Grossman-Alexander, M. (1998). The view from the road: Implications for stress recovery and immunization. *Journal of Environmental Psychology, 18*(2), 113–140.

Pati, D., Harvey, T. E. Jr., & Barach, P. (2008). Relationships between exterior views and nurse stress: An exploratory examination. *Health Environments Research & Design Journal, 1*(2), 27–38.

Pilcher, E. J., Newman, P., & Manning, R. E. (2009). Understanding and managing experiential aspects of soundscapes at Muir Woods National Monument. *Environmental Management*, *43*(3), 425–435.

Pretty, J. (2004). How nature contributes to mental and physical health. *Spirituality and Health International*, *5*(2), 68–78.

Pretty, J., Peacock, J., Sellens, M., & Griffin, M. (2005). The mental and physical health outcomes of green exercise. *International Journal of Environmental Health Research*, *15*(5), 319–337.

Raanaas, R. K., Evensen, K. H., Rich, D., Sjøstrøm, G., & Patil, G. (2011). Benefits of indoor plants on attention capacity in an office setting. *Journal of Environmental Psychology*, *31*(1), 99–105.

Ratcliffe, E., Gatersleben, B., & Sowden, P. T. (2013). Bird sounds and their contributions to perceived attention restoration and stress recovery. *Journal of Environmental Psychology*, *36*, 221–228.

Ratcliffe, E., Gatersleben, B., & Sowden, P. T. (2016). Associations with bird sounds: How do they relate to perceived restorative potential? *Journal of Environmental Psychology*, *47*, 136–144.

Roe, J. J., Thompson, C. W., Aspinall, P. A., Brewer, M. J., Duff, E. I., Miller, D., Mitchell, R., & Clow, A. (2013). Green space and stress: Evidence from cortisol measures in deprived urban communities. *International Journal of Environmental Research and Public Health*, *10*(9), 4086–4103.

Rojas-Rueda, D., Nieuwenhuijsen, M. J., Gascon, M., Perez-Leon, D., & Mudu, P. (2019). Green spaces and mortality: A systematic review and meta-analysis of cohort studies. *The Lancet Planetary Health*, *3*(11), e469–e477.

Ruggles, D. H. (2017). *Beauty, neuroscience & architecture*. Fibonacci, LLC.

Rybczynski, W. (1999). *A clearing in the distance: Frederick Law Olmsted and America in the nineteenth century*. Scribner.

Schroeder, H. W. (1991). The psychological value of trees. *The Public Garden: Journal of the American Association of Botanical Gardens and Arboreta*, 6.

Shin, J. C., Parab, K. V., An, R., & Grigsby-Toussaint, D. S. (2020). Greenspace exposure and sleep: A systematic review. *Environmental Research*, *182*, 109081.

Soga, M., Gaston, K. J., & Yamaura, Y. (2017). Gardening is beneficial for health: A meta-analysis. *Preventive Medicine Reports*, *5*, 92–99.

Squire, D. (2002). *The healing garden: Natural healing for mind, body and soul*. Robson Books Limited.

Stevenson, E. (1977). *Park maker: A life of Frederick Law Olmsted*. Transaction Publishers.

Stevenson, M. P., Dewhurst, R., Schilhab, T., & Bentsen, P. (2019). Cognitive restoration in children following exposure to nature: Evidence from the attention network task and mobile eye tracking. *Frontiers in Psychology*, *10*, 42. https://doi.org/10.3389/fpsyg.2019.00042

Stigsdotter, U. A., & Grahn, P. (2004). A garden at your workplace may reduce stress. *Design & Health*, 147–157.

Stigsdotter, U. K., Ekholm, O., Schipperijn, J., Toftager, M., Kamper-Jørgensen, F., & Randrup, T. B. (2010). Health promoting outdoor environments—Associations between green space, and health, health-related quality of life and stress based on a Danish national representative survey. *Scandinavian Journal of Public Health*, *38*(4), 411–417.

Stephen, S. R. (1993). Introduction. In Wilson, E.O. & Kellert, S. R. (Eds.). *The biophilia hypothesis*. Island Press, 20–30.

Su, J. G., Dadvand, P., Nieuwenhuijsen, M. J., Bartoll, X., & Jerrett, M. (2019). Associations of green space metrics with health and behavior outcomes at different buffer sizes and remote sensing sensor resolutions. *Environment International*, *126*, 162–170.

Sugaya, S., Kasetani, T., Qiu-Ji, Z., Guo, W. Z., Udagawa, A., Nomura, J., Sugita, K., Ohta, R., & Suzuki, N. (2011). Studies on the amounts of serum hydroperoxide, MMP-3, urinary 8-OHdG, and salivary IgA in rheumatoid arthritis patients who experienced shinrin-yoku (forest-air bathing and walking). *Chiba Medical Journal*, *87*(5), 181–188.

Szczygiel, B., & Hewitt, R. (2000). Nineteenth-century medical landscapes: John H. Rauch, Frederick Law Olmsted, and the search for salubrity. *Bulletin of Anesthesia History*, *19*(2), 27–28.

Szczygiel, B., & Hewitt, R. (2000). Nineteenth-century medical landscapes: John H. Rauch, Frederick Law Olmsted, and the search for salubrity. *Bulletin of the History of Medicine*, *74*(4), 708–734.

Taylor, A. F., Kuo, F. E., & Sullivan, W. C. (2002). Views of nature and self-discipline: Evidence from inner city children. *Journal of Environmental Psychology*, *22*(1–2), 49–63.

Thompson, J. D., & Goldin, G. (1975). *The hospital: A social and architectural history*. Yale University Press.

Thompson, C. W., Roe, J., Aspinall, P., Mitchell, R., Clow, A., & Miller, D. (2012). More green space is linked to less stress in deprived communities: Evidence from salivary cortisol patterns. *Landscape and Urban Planning*, *105*(3), 221–229.

Twohig-Bennett, C., & Jones, A. (2018). The health benefits of the great outdoors: A systematic review and meta-analysis of greenspace exposure and health outcomes. *Environmental Research*, *166*, 628–637.

Ulrich, R. S. (1977). Visual landscape preference: A model and application. *Man-Environment Systems*, *7*, 279–293.

Ulrich, R. S. (1979). Visual landscapes and psychological well-being. *Landscape Research*, *4*(1), 17–23.

Ulrich, R. S. (1983). Aesthetic and affective response to natural environment. In I. Altman, & J. F. Wohlwill (Eds.), *Human behavior and environment: Advances in theory and research* (Vol. 6; pp. 85–125). Plenum.

Ulrich, R. S. (1984). View through a window may influence recovery from surgery. *Science*, 224(4647), 420–421.

Ulrich, R. S. (1993). Biophilia, biophobia, and natural landscapes. In S. R. Keller, & E. O. Wilson (Eds.), *The biophilia hypothesis* (pp. 73–137)). Island Press.

Ulrich, R. S. (1999). Effects of gardens on health outcomes: Theory and research. In Cooper-Marcus, C., & Barnes, M. (Eds.), *Healing gardens: Therapeutic benefits and design recommendations*. John Wiley & Sons.

Ulrich, R. S., Simons, R. F., Losito, B. D., Fiorito, E., Miles, M. A., & Zelson, M. (1991). Stress recovery during exposure to natural and urban environments. *Journal of Environmental Psychology*, *11*(3), 201–230.

Van den Berg, A. E., Koole, S. L., & van der Wulp, N. Y. (2003). Environmental preference and restoration:(How) are they related? *Journal of Environmental Psychology*, *23*(2), 135–146.

Vanaken, G. J., & Danckaerts, M. (2018). Impact of green space exposure on children's and adolescents' mental health: A systematic review. *International Journal of Environmental Research and Public Health, 15*(12), 2668.

Verderber, S. (2010). *Innovations in hospital architecture.* Routledge.

Vincent, E., Battisto, D., Grimes, L., & McCubbin, J. (2010). The effects of nature images on pain in a simulated hospital patient room. *Health Environments Research & Design Journal, 3*(3), 42–55.

Voelker, S., & Kistemann, T. (2013). Reprint of: "I'm always entirely happy when I'm here!" Urban blue enhancing human health and well-being in Cologne and Düsseldorf, *Germany. Social Science & Medicine, 91,* 141–152.

Walker, S. E., & Duffield, B. S. (1983). Urban parks and open spaces—An overview. *Landscape Research, 8*(2), 2–12.

Wang, R., Zhao, J., Meitner, M. J., Hu, Y., & Xu, X. (2019). Characteristics of urban green spaces in relation to aesthetic preference and stress recovery. *Urban Forestry & Urban Greening, 41,* 6–13.

Ward, W. E. (1952). The lotus symbol: Its meaning in Buddhist art and philosophy. *The Journal of Aesthetics and Art Criticism, 11*(2), 135–146.

Ward-Thompson, C. (2011). Linking landscape and health: The recurring theme. *Landscape and Urban Planning, 99*(3), 187–195.

Williams, A. (1998). Therapeutic landscapes in holistic medicine. *Social Science & Medicine, 46*(9), 1193–1203.

Williams, A. (Ed.). (1999). *Therapeutic landscapes: The dynamic between place and wellness.* University Press of America.

Wilson, E. O. (1993). Biophilia and the conservation ethics. In Wilson, E.O. & Kellert, S. R. (Eds.). *The biophilia hypothesis.* Island Press, 31–41.

Yaniv, Z., & Bachrach, U. (2005). *Handbook of medicinal plants.* Food Products Press.

Yeager, R. A., Smith, T. R., & Bhatnagar, A. (2020). Green environments and cardiovascular health. *Trends in Cardiovascular Medicine, 30*(4), 241–246.

Zajonc, R. B. (1980). Feeling and thinking: Preferences need no inferences. *American Psychologist, 35,* 151–175.

3 Reconnect People and Nature through Windows in Healthcare Environments

Windows seem to be the primary means of providing a connection between urban dwellers and nature. A national survey by the Environmental Protection Agency (EPA) found that the average American spends around 87% of their life in enclosed buildings and about 6% of their life in enclosed vehicles (Klepeis et al., 2001). Window views are deemed as necessities in the maintenance of a healthy life—not merely in terms of the absence of disease or infirmity, but also for a state of complete physical, mental, and social well-being (World Health Organization, 1946). This chapter first summarizes the effects of windows and the lack of windows, in everyday amenities, including homes, schools, and workplaces. It then discusses the health benefits/outcomes of windows in healthcare environments, particularly window views of nature and daylight.

Effects of Windows and No Windows

Windowed versus Windowless Environments

The report *A Room with a View* by the Institute for Research in Construction (National Research Council Canada) thoroughly reviewed scientific studies from a variety of disciplines examining the effects of windowed and windowless environments on schooling, work, and everyday life and well-being (Farley & Veitch, 2001). Early systematic reviews of people's reactions to windows were conducted in response to energy conservation trends in the building design system of the 1970s (Collins, 1975; Keep, 1977). Along with the advancement of artificial lighting and mechanical ventilation, it was thought that the reduction of window sizes or the complete elimination of windows would lead to substantial energy savings (Farley & Veitch, 2001). However, Collins' (1975) extensive literature review demonstrated that, beyond light and air, windows provide more functions and benefits for people: Windows provide a view to the outside; knowledge of the weather and time of day; relief from feelings of claustrophobia, monotony, or boredom; and a change of focus as well as adding beauty to a room and serving as an indicator of estate and wealth. In the case of healthcare buildings, windows

DOI: 10.4324/9781003122180-3

and daylight are perceived to have a profound value other than simply for energy saving (Baker & Steemers, 2013).

Windows as micro-restorative settings provide extensive psychological and health benefits (Kaplan, 2001). The lack of windows or natural daylight results in the absence of cues about the natural world, which in itself is a form of sensory deprivation and can be extremely detrimental to human beings (Boubekri, 2014). A windowless residential environment tends to generate very negative reactions among occupants. Generally, a strong desire for windows exists among students and parents in the school environment as well as workers in offices and factories (Collins, 1975). Windows have also been linked to certain behavioral characteristics. Studies have shown that window views of nature near the home can help children concentrate, inhibit impulse behaviors, and lead more effective, self-disciplined (Taylor et al., 2002). Residents in apartments with window views of nature tend to demonstrate less aggressive behaviors and violence than those with no nature views (Kuo & Sullivan, 2001).

In addition, a windowed office room was found to be significantly more motivating than a windowless one in a work environment with respect to improving employees' overall satisfaction with their job and workplace, reducing physical and psychological discomfort, promoting office employees' business performance as well as their working memory and ability to concentrate, enhancing mood, and improving their qualities of after-work life (Aries et al., 2010; Boubekri & Haghighat, 1993; Boubekri et al., 2014; Dravigne et al., 2008; Ko et al., 2020; Leather et al., 1998; Nagy et al., 1995; Stone, 1998). In environments where window access is unavailable, occupants tend to compensate with the use of nature-themed visual decorations or indoor plants (Bringslimark et al., 2009; Dijkstra et al., 2008; Heerwagen & Orians, 1986; Lankston et al., 2010; Nanda et al., 2011; Park & Mattson, 2009). Stone and Irvine (1994) conducted a study that explored different task types and window access in a work environment. They found that window access in the room tended to be more effective for creative tasks than monotonous tasks such as filling and computation; moreover, boredom tended to be reduced when one worked while facing the window. For windowed environments, the varying sizes of the windows, distances to the windows, and content and characteristics of window views all led to different outcomes.

Window Attributes

Size and Shape of Windows

An early investigation by Ne'Eman and Hopkinson (1970) examined how the various factors affected people's judgment on a minimum size of the window and concluded that the lighting conditions, both indoors and through the window, as well as the solar angle throughout the day and the sky luminance seemed not to be the main factors impacting the appraisal of the minimum size of window. Generally, participants preferred wider windows for views of nearer objects; increasing the window width and the number of windows within the limits of a horizontal viewing angle of 60° were favored and effective. The researchers also estimated that the minimum acceptable window width was 2.2–3.2 m, and the window width was directly proportional to the distance between the viewer and the window (window width over distance from the window was constant for any viewing point). In order to obtain a satisfying window size, the window should occupy no less than 35% of the window wall. A similar study confirmed that wider windows were generally preferred than the taller ones, and windows occupying 10% or less of the window wall were regarded as extremely unsatisfactory (Farley & Veitch, 2001; Keighley, 1973).

Butler and Steuerwald (1991) conducted two experiments and concluded that window shape, room size and esthetics of window views have substantial effects on window size preferences. Participants preferred shapes of windows that were proportional to the shape of the window wall, as determined by the room size. Nearly square windows were preferred for small rooms (which had a square wall) whereas very wide windows were preferred for large rooms (which had rectangular walls). Beautiful window views, such as scenes of a wooded area or a mountain, impacted the preferences for window size and the height of windowsills: Larger windows and lower sills were generally preferred for beautiful sciences to capture the "whole" view, regardless of the size of the room.

Dogrusoy and Tureyen (2007) found similar conclusions. Among six shapes and layouts of office windows with the same views, employees preferred their individual workspaces to be closer to the full-height window wall (i.e., curtain wall), and horizontal window stripes were largely preferred, followed by horizontally arranged square-shaped windows. Narrow, rectangular windows, vertical windows, and round windows were the least preferred. The top ranked factors when determining window preferences were natural lighting and sunlight, natural ventilation, a sense of spaciousness, noise buffering, and mood enhancement (Dogrusoy & Tureyen, 2007).

Distances to the Window

People generally prefer to stay closer to windows. A greater distance to windows was found to be associated with lower perceived pleasantness, adequacy, and satisfaction of the view (Cooper et al., 1973). A viewer further from the window tends to prefer a wider and larger window to perceive a quality view. However, the distance between the viewer and the nearest window seemed not to influence the viewer's estimation of the daylight illuminance. In fact, people tended to overestimate the proportion of daylight that they worked based on their distance from the windows; meanwhile, estimates about daylight levels depended on psychological considerations, such as the judgment of apparent brightness distribution and the preference for the window view (Galasiu & Veitch, 2006; Wells, 1965). One experiment observed office workers' seating preference and their control of the office lighting and found that workstations located near the window were the most appreciated by participants even though they worked on computer tasks. When the distance between the workstation and the window increased, more participants chose to add extra electric light despite the adequacy of the total interior illuminance (Laurentin et al., 1998).

Content and Quality of Window Views

Views of Nature versus Built Environments

Kaplan (1993) found that the content of the window view is more important than simply having a window. Numerous studies have shown that window views of nature are preferred over built environments. Window views of other buildings, parking lots, and urban streets generally contribute limited restoration (Kaplan, 1993; Ulrich, 1984). Window views of nature from home play a significant role with respect to effective functioning and behaviors as compared to no views or views of urban scenes. Researchers found that residents in apartments with window views of nature demonstrated less aggressive behaviors and violence than those with no nature views (Kuo & Sullivan, 2001). Window views from home influence residents' satisfaction with the residential environment as well as the neighborhood (Kaplan, 2001; Kearney, 2006). Cooper Marcus and Sarkissian (1986) emphasized views from windows in residential design as most residents tended to judge the attractiveness of their neighborhood simply by what they can see from their windows. People prefer a visual diversity that "includes a distant open view, a closer view of greenery, and some human activity" (p. 47).

Employees working in an office building reported that window views of trees and distant hills were significantly more favorable than nearby buildings and views of the sky (Markus, 1967). Window views of natural scenes, such as the forest, trees, vegetation, plants, and foliage, were found to be effective in reducing job-related stress and improving job satisfaction (Leather et al., 1998; Sop Shin, 2007). Lottrup and colleagues (2012) examined six companies in Sweden with a total of 402 participants who have views and access to the outside. The results revealed that window views dominated by the sky, trees, flowers, and park-like environments were associated with higher satisfaction with the workspace than views described as cars/traffic, mowed lawns, and wild nature. Window views of buildings/signs or no views were the least preferred by the employees. Lottrup and colleagues (2012) further found a significant relationship between view satisfaction and the job ability: Respondents who reported "high view satisfaction" had significantly higher odds for reporting "high work ability" than respondents who reported "low/medium view satisfaction" (p. 11).

Complexity of Window Views

As Kaplan and Wendt (1972) indicated, window views judged as complex generally gained the highest preference, and complex nature scenes were preferred to urban scenes that are equivalent in complexity. These findings are further proven by the attention-restoration theory. Butler and Steuerwald (1991) made similar conclusions that one important aspect of the beauty/preference of nature-oriented window views was complexity. Most natural views are relatively complex, meaning they are not too simple or too overwhelming, due to the fractal-like geometry of natural elements. Kaplan (1993) also suggested that the optimum window views should include more rather than fewer natural features that have both coherence (distinct grouping of elements) and focus (some contrasting elements that captures the viewer's attention).

Windows and Natural Daylight

A major function of windows is to provide natural daylight. Although artificial lighting in a windowless room does not seem to affect people's work performance, some hypotheses have even favored a windowless room to reduce distractions on certain tasks (Stone, 1998). In addition, participants from various studies have claimed that windows are important environmental features, and they preferred natural daylight as their primary source of lighting (Haans, 2014; Veitch et al., 1993). Natural daylight through windows has been shown to be important for physiological and psychological well-being. Boubekri (2008, 2014) thoroughly analyzed the health benefits of natural daylight in his two books about daylighting design, architecture, and health. A relatively new branch of medicine, chronotherapy, has been developed to facilitate treatments for modern people's sicknesses, particularly when they lack natural daylight (Czeisler et al., 1981).

Natural daylight has been closely tied to two important health issues: vitamin D deficiency and illnesses resulting from it, and people's diurnal circadian rhythm and related depression (Boubekri, 2014). A windowless environment can significantly reduce the hours of exposure to natural daylight and sunlight, thereby leading to a sequence of hormonal disorders. Exposure to sunlight produces the major proportion of vitamin D required by the human body and serves as a catalyst for the secretion of serotonin, a hormone responsible for people's state of alertness (Boubekri, 2014; Glerup et al., 2000). Daylight–darkness cycling helps maintain the balance between serotonin and melatonin levels, regulate circadian rhythms and sleep patterns, and maintain the functioning and balance of vital signs, energy, and circulation in the human body (Boubekri, 2014). Populations living in northern latitudes frequently experience seasonal depression symptoms, referred to as seasonal affective disorder. Küller and Lindsten (1992) investigated Swedish adolescents' body growth and hormone patterns in windowed and windowless classrooms and found that the absence of daylight might have delayed the annual variations in the production of the stress hormone cortisol by as much as two months for children in windowless classrooms, which in turn influenced sociability and the ability to concentrate.

Natural daylight also influences people's psychological and mental health status in the work environment. Sunlight penetration through windows in a workplace has direct effects on improving workers' emotional response and appraisal of job satisfaction while reducing their intention to quit (Boubekri et al., 1991; Leather et al., 1998). More specifically, sitting sideways to the window receiving sunlight penetration resulted in people being significantly more relaxed than when sitting facing the window (Boubekri et al., 1991). Küller and Wetterberg (1996) compared subterranean work environments with those above ground and found that spaces below the ground level were perceived as more enclosed and having lighting conditions that they considered less bright and pleasant. Employees working in subterranean spaces complained more frequently about visual fatigue and noise. Hormonal patterns also varied between employees in under- and above-ground work environments: The level of morning cortisol showed substantial annual variations among those who worked above ground but was much less pronounced among those who worked below ground. The concentration and diurnal variation of melatonin were also much larger for people working in subterranean environments.

Visual and Thermal Comfort

Light, direct sunlight particularly, is not merely related to the visual experience but is strongly connected to the thermal qualities and sensorial characteristics of a space, directly impacting on air movement and surface temperatures (Baker & Steemers, 2013). Although not the focus of this chapter, it is worth mentioning some negative impacts of windows when the shading structure was not properly designed. Depending on the size, orientation, and solar shading configuration, a window could impact occupants' visual and thermal comfort and is directly linked to the energy consumption of the building (Shikder et al., 2010). Although window seats are generally preferred, being close to a window and rating the lighting as being of lower quality can result in utility problems, such as glares and thermal discomfort (Aries et al., 2010). Similarly, Veitch and colleagues (2005) found that a greater window distance was associated with fewer glare or heat problems in open-plan building environments. Controversial conclusions were generated from field studies that intensive daylighting was associated with frequent complaints of sun and glare, which were thus considered unpleasant in some office buildings (Galasiu & Veitch, 2006). A high-performance, insulated glazing system will generally admit more daylight and less heat than a typical window, allowing for daylighting without negatively impacting the building cooling load in the summer (Ander & US Department of Energy, 2016).

Above all, a daylighting-optimized fenestration design will increase system performance. The windows for daylight delivery should have a glazing with a very high visible light transmittance (VLT), and the windows for views should have a relatively low VLT to prevent glare. In fact, the higher the window head height, the deeper into the space the daylight can penetrate; therefore, good daylighting fenestration practices suggest two discrete types of window components: a daylight window system and a view window system (Ander & US Department of Energy, 2016).

Windows, Views, and Daylight in Healthcare Environments

Windows in Healthcare Environments

For patients stressed by disease or illness, flourishing natural scenes with blue and green hues could induce a state of calm and positively affect their mood (Lankston et al., 2010). For certain fragile patients who are not allowed outside, windowside may be the most approachable place allowing them to communicate with the external world. For healthcare providers and staff members working longer shifts in hospitals (shifts of 12 hours or longer are common for nurses in the US), a windowless workspace could be extremely depressing and thus negatively impact the care that patients receive and the well-being of the staff members (Stimpfel et al., 2012). An important topic of discussion has focused on enhancing the qualities of healthcare environments through user-centered design; therefore, people–nature engagement and window-themed studies have attracted continuous research effort in the realm of healthcare design since the 1970s (Jiang et al., 2017; Raanaas et al., 2012; Ulrich, 1984; Verderber, 1986; Wilson, 1972).

Window Effects for Patients

As early as the 1970s, a group of scholars were drawn to the topics of hospital windows. Keep and colleagues (1980) compared two groups of patients who had survived a stay of at least 48 hours in the windowed versus windowless intensive therapy units (ITUs) in Norwich, England. Patients from the windowless ITU had a less accurate memory of the length of their stay and were less oriented in time during their stay. Patients in the windowless ITU experienced twice as many hallucinations and delusions as those in the windowed ITU. The seminal study by Roger Ulrich (1984) examined inpatients' recovery situation after the same cholecystectomy surgery in a suburban Pennsylvania hospital between 1972 and 1981. Twenty-three pairs of patients' medical records during the hospitalization period were analyzed to determine whether the patient room with a window view of trees might have better restorative effects than the room with a view of a brick wall. The results indicated that, compared to the wall-view group, patients with the tree view had shorter postoperative hospital stays, received fewer negative evaluation comments from nurses, took fewer moderate and strong analgesic doses, and had slightly fewer complications from postoperative conditions such as headache and nausea.

Verderber (1986) conducted a sophisticated study that investigated a series of healthcare spaces ranging from highly windowed to windowless as well as the relationship between a broad spectrum of window attributes and respondents' cognitive and behavioral responses. Photo questionnaires were administered to 125 staff members and 125 inpatients at physical medicine and rehabilitation (PMR) units across six hospitals in Chicago. A total of 64 photographs in the questionnaire sampled the patient rooms, treatment rooms, and staff offices of 11 PMR units with different levels of windowness and window attributes, including view content, daylight, sill height, screens, and aperture size. According to the results, the most desired views from therapy rooms were of trees and lawns, the surrounding neighborhood, and people outside. Windows with high sills from the floor, distant from the viewer, and views obscured by nearby walls, screens, or furnishings were rated as insufficient windowness and nearly equivalent to having no window views at all. The quality of the window views was found to be directly influential on respondents' overall satisfaction with the hospital environment. Based on the same fieldwork sites, Verderber and Reuman (1987) further investigated windows and the impacts on occupants' states of well-being. Patients were found to be more negatively impacted by poorly windowed rooms, compared to staff members; in addition, paralyzed, immobile, and visually impaired patients as well as minority patients were more susceptible to windows at a greater distance (more than 10 feet) for long hours per day or in rooms with limited view information content.

Among the few studies using a real patient sample in a real healthcare facility, Raanaas and colleagues (2012) explored the health benefits of windows and natural views in a residential rehabilitation center. The researchers randomly assigned 278 coronary and pulmonary patients to a patient room with a panoramic view of natural surroundings or with a view either partially or entirely blocked by buildings. Patients in the room with a panoramic view showed the greatest improvement in mental and physical health and the overall satisfaction during the rehabilitation program, although the degree of improvement varied by gender and diagnosis. Patients with a panoramic view to nature also reported using the room as "a place to withdraw to a greater extent" and the place to stay when they wanted to be alone (Raanaas et al., 2012, p. 30) (Figure 3.1).

A few studies generated some indirect evidence using either simulated patients or simulated healthcare environments to support the health benefits of window views. Vincent and colleagues (2010a, 2010b) used a simulated patient room (a true scale mock-up) with different views of nature. Pain was induced through a cold pressor task that required participants to immerse their hands in ice water for up to 120 seconds. Their results revealed that participants with natural views representing prospect-refuge

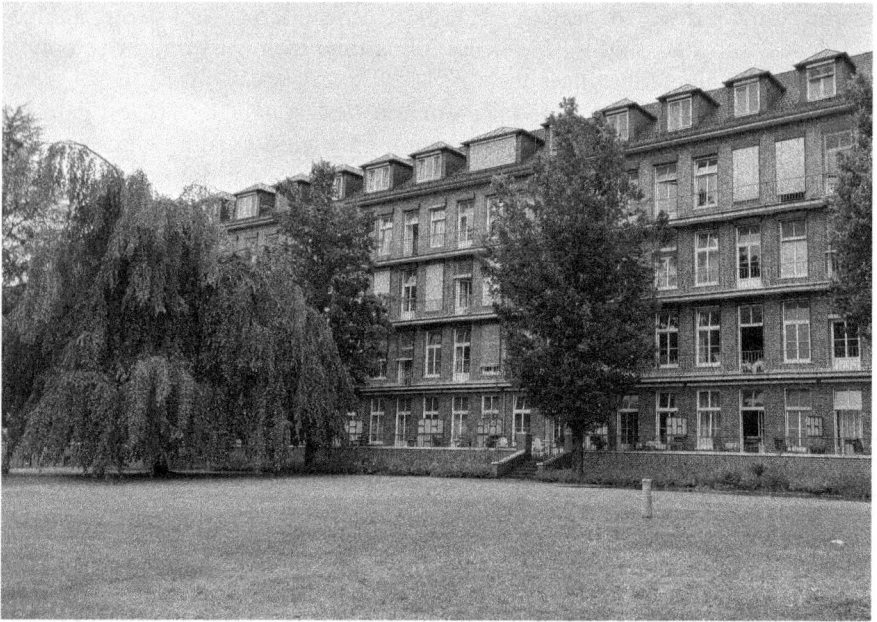

Figure 3.1 Large, operable windows facing to a green open space at the old patient room building of Klinikum Oldenburg, Oldenburg, Germany; the hospital was built in the early 20th century

Source: © Austin Ferguson at Heinle, Wischer und Partner

perceived the lowest level of sensory pain, whereas the control group with no views perceived the highest level of sensory pain. Jiang's (2015) and Jiang and colleagues' (2017) studies simulated a hospital waiting room with different types of window views. Participants were exposed to a thrilling video at the beginning of the study to induce their physiological status (i.e., blood pressure and heart rate) as a simulation of the stressful status. The results revealed that the restorative effects of window views increased along with the increased transparency of window views to nature. This study will be discussed in greater depth in a later chapter of the book.

Window Effects for Staff

Stress has been frequently ranked as a top job-related concern among healthcare professionals, particularly nurses (Burton et al., 2017; Hofmann, 2018; O'Dowd et al., 2018). The American Nursing Association has conducted two national surveys, in 2001 and 2011, to explore nurses' concerns about health and safety in their work environments. The top two health and safety concerns according to 4,614 nurses in 2011 were stress and overwork (74%) and disabling musculoskeletal injury (62%), which remained the same since the 2001 survey (American Nursing Association, 2011). In a cross-sectional study, the physical environment of the workplace was ranked as a major cause of job stress in nurses (Najimi et al., 2012). However, many spaces in large hospitals lack sufficient window views and natural daylight, which could add weights to environmental stressors. Working in these spaces, such as the centralized nursing station, radiology unit, operating rooms, and many other clinical support rooms located deep in the building block, could result in a deprivation of nature contact. A significant proportion of nurses reported having zero hour exposure to an external view throughout their entire shift (Pati et al., 2008).

In an examination of the window effects on healthcare professionals, several studies have suggested the need to incorporate windows into work environments to help reduce work-related stress and burnouts. Pati and colleagues (2008) explored the relationships between exterior views and nurse stress and alertness through a mixed-method study. Two hospitals in the Atlanta metropolitan area were chosen as the fieldwork sites, and a small sample of nurses participated in the study. Nurses' chronic stress and their acute stress and alertness before and after a 12-hour shift were measured using different questionnaires. The results revealed an association between window view attributes and nurses' acute stress. The duration of window views and alertness and stress is conditional on the exterior view content, indicating the mediating effect of natural views in nurses' alertness retention and stress reduction as compared to other types of views (Pati et al., 2008).

Zadeh and colleagues (2014) investigated the impacts of windows and daylight on nurses' physiological, psychological, and behavioral health in an acute care unit of a community hospital in Texas. Nurses working at two clusters of nurse stations in the same patient ward were compared; one had no windows or access to daylight and the other had windows that looked out on portions of the hospital building, the sky, and a courtyard. The findings indicated that the window and daylight group of nurses tended to experience lower blood pressure and higher blood oxygen saturation; both communication and laughter increased while subsidiary behavior indicators of sleepiness and deteriorated mood decreased for the window and daylight group, which were in line with the micro-restorative effect of windows and daylight in existing literature.

Natural Daylight in Healthcare Environments

Natural Daylight for Patients

Large skylights were not rare in early hospitals. For example, Pennsylvania Hospital—the oldest hospital in the US, built in 1751—had large skylights in the middle of the roof on the original building as surgical operations were timed to coincide with the passage of the sun across the skylights (Vinall, 1997). Nurses and doctors have recognized natural daylight as an important element in patient rooms to aid in assessing patient recovery by recognizing and interpreting changes in patient skin color (Alzubaidi et al., 2013). Today's hospitals have replaced natural daylight with advanced artificial lighting for surgical and many other tasks. However, such environments lacking light periodicity could lead to a lost track of circadian rhythms and many other disorders among hospital occupants. According to many studies, bedridden patients and populations with limited mobilities were found having very low levels of vitamin D in winter, which is directly related to the prolonged indoor stay and a lack of sufficient sunlight (Boubekri, 2014). Vitamin D deficiency is typical among ICU patients and has been found to be associated with longer time to ICU discharge and a trend toward increased risk of ICU-acquired infection (Higgins et al., 2012).

Shepley and colleagues (2012) investigated the impacts of window views and daylight on ICU patients and identified trends, although not statistically significant, suggesting that increased light levels and natural views could reduce patients' pain perception and length of stay. In contrast, some studies have concluded that the presence of a window in an ICU room did not improve outcomes for patients with critical conditions. Wunsch and colleagues (2011) studied seven neurological ICU rooms with or without windows at a hospital in New York and compared the recovery progress at hospital discharge, 3 months, and 1 year for 789 patients randomly assigned to the ICU rooms from 1997 to 2006. No statistically significant differences were identified between patients in windowed or windowless ICU rooms regarding the degree of disability/dependence scores and any secondary outcomes, including the recovery progress, ICU and hospital length of stay, and mortality rate.

Natural daylight has been found to be effective in reducing regular inpatients' length of hospital stay. In a study conducted in a hospital in Incheon, Korea, 1,167 inpatients' data of length of hospital stays were investigated regarding the different levels of daylight and illuminance in the patient rooms (Choi et al., 2012). The results indicated that patients' average length of stay in single-bed patient rooms oriented to the southeast (which remain brighter and have much higher illuminance across all seasons) was significantly shorter than those in rooms oriented to the northwest. High illuminance in the morning seemed to be more beneficial than in the afternoon, and visual discomfort caused by excessive daylight and glare can be prevented by installing proper shading devices, such as vertical or horizontal blinds, and shading structures controllable by patients may have a positive effect on patients' physiological and psychological conditions (Choi et al., 2012). In another study comparing patients' length of hospital stay in multi-bed patient rooms in a general hospital, patients assigned to the windowside beds were found to have significantly shorter lengths of stays than those assigned to the beds next to the door (farthest from the window) based on 33,921 pairs of participants' hospitalization data (Park et al., 2018).

For other groups of patients, natural daylight has been found to be beneficial to patients' psychological, emotional, and behavioral health and well-being.

Beauchemin and Hays (1996) found that patients hospitalized for severe depression reduced their length of stay by an average of 2.6 days if assigned to a sunny patient room rather than a dull room overlooking spaces in shadow. Sufficient daylight has also been found to be specifically associated with reduced depression for pregnant women (Oren et al., 2002). In Eldaly and colleagues' (2016) study about daylight sufficiency in psychiatric hospital wards and patient satisfaction, many positive relationships were found between daylight intensity and patients' satisfaction toward healthcare services, life enjoyment, and the visual and thermal comfort of the physical environment. To note that, this study was conducted on an Egyptian sample and indicated a desire for sufficient daylight even in a representative geolocation categorized as having a high intensity of solar radiation (Omran, 2000). Similarly, a survey of nurses and doctors in a hospital in Doha, Qatar, rated sufficient daylight in a patient room as a potential facilitator in patient recovery (Alzubaidi et al., 2013).

Natural Daylight for Staff

Healthcare providers often rank the availability of daylight and adequate illumination as the top factors in their perception of the design quality of hospitals' physical environments (Mourshed & Zhao, 2012). A nurse's notes for a report on hospital design in England mentioned that "it makes you happier to be working in a nice environment, pleasant view, sufficient daylight and the possibility of opening a window for fresh air" (Rechel et al., 2009, p. 1027). In a study of two ICUs with or without windows and natural daylight in New Hampshire, staff members' absenteeism and staff vacancy were found to be significantly correlated to window views and natural light: Both average vacancy rate and absenteeism per person decreased in the ICU with high levels of natural light and window views (Shepley et al., 2012). A study using a sample of 141 nurses who worked in a university hospital in Antalya, Turkey, indicated that daylight exposure during work impacted nurses' work-related stress and job satisfaction. Exposure to daylight for at least 3 hours per day was found to cause less stress and higher satisfaction at work (Alimoglu & Donmez, 2005). The systematic investigation of daylight's therapeutic effects in the healthcare context can be found in literature review studies conducted by Joarder et al. (2009) as well as Behringer's (2011) thesis about daylight in healthcare design.

References

Alimoglu, M. K., & Donmez, L. (2005). Daylight exposure and the other predictors of burnout among nurses in a university hospital. *International Journal of Nursing Studies*, *42*(5), 549–555.

Alzubaidi, S., Roaf, S., Banfill, P. F. G., Talib, R. A., & Al-Ansari, A. (2013). Survey of hospitals lighting: Daylight and staff preferences. *International Journal of Energy Engineering*, *3*(6), 287–293.

American Nursing Association. (2011). 2011 ANA Health and Safety Survey. https://www.nursingworld.org/practice-policy/work-environment/health-safety/health-safety-survey/

Ander, G. D. & U.S. Department of Energy. (2016). Daylighting. Whole Building Design Guide. https://www.wbdg.org/resources/daylighting

Aries, M. B., Veitch, J. A., & Newsham, G. R. (2010). Windows, view, and office characteristics predict physical and psychological discomfort. *Journal of Environmental Psychology, 30*(4), 533–541.

Baker, N., & Steemers, K. (2013). *Daylight design of buildings: A handbook for architects and engineers.* Taylor & Francis.

Beauchemin, K. M., & Hays, P. (1996). Sunny hospital rooms expedite recovery from severe and refractory depressions. *Journal of Affective Disorders, 40*(1–2), 49–51.

Behringer, E. (2011). The daylight imperative. All Theses. 1120. https://tigerprints.clemson.edu/all_theses/1120

Boubekri, M. (2008). *Daylighting, architecture and health: Building design strategies.* Routledge.

Boubekri, M. (2014). *Daylighting design: Planning strategies and best practice solutions.* Birkhäuser.

Boubekri, M., Cheung, I. N., Reid, K. J., Wang, C. H., & Zee, P. C. (2014). Impact of windows and daylight exposure on overall health and sleep quality of office workers: A case-control pilot study. *Journal of Clinical Sleep Medicine, 10*(6), 603–611.

Boubekri, M., & Haghighat, F. (1993). Windows and environmental satisfaction: A survey study of an office building. *Indoor Environment, 2*(3), 164–172.

Boubekri, M., Hull, R. B., & Boyer, L. L. (1991). Impact of window size and sunlight penetration on office workers' mood and satisfaction: A novel way of assessing sunlight. *Environment and Behavior, 23*(4), 474–493.

Bringslimark, T., Hartig, T., & Patil, G. G. (2009). The psychological benefits of indoor plants: A critical review of the experimental literature. *Journal of Environmental Psychology, 29*(4), 422–433.

Burton, A., Burgess, C., Dean, S., Koutsopoulou, G. Z., & Hugh-Jones, S. (2017). How effective are mindfulness-based interventions for reducing stress among healthcare professionals? A systematic review and meta-analysis. *Stress and Health, 33*(1), 3–13.

Butler, D. L., & Steuerwald, B. L. (1991). Effects of view and room size on window size preferences made in models. *Environment and Behavior, 23*(3), 334–358.

Choi, J. H., Beltran, L. O., & Kim, H. S. (2012). Impacts of indoor daylight environments on patient average length of stay (ALOS) in a healthcare facility. *Building and Environment, 50*, 65–75.

Collins, B. L. (1975). *Windows and people: A literature survey. Psychological reaction to environments with and without windows.* National Bureau of Standards.

Cooper, J. R., Wiltshire, T. J., & Hardy, A. C. (1973). Attitudes towards the use of heat rejecting/low light transmission glasses in office buildings. *Proceedings of CIE conference, Istanbul, on "Windows and their function in architectural design."*

Cooper Marcus, C., & Sarkissian, W. (1986). *Housing as if people mattered: Site design guidelines for the planning of medium-density family housing* (Vol. 4). University of California Press.

Czeisler, C. A., Richardson, G. S., Coleman, R. M., Zimmerman, J. C., Moore-Ede, M. C., Dement, W. C., & Weitzman, E. D. (1981). Chronotherapy: Resetting the circadian clocks of patients with delayed sleep phase insomnia. *Sleep, 4*(1), 1–21.

Dijkstra, K., Pieterse, M. E., & Pruyn, A. (2008). Stress-reducing effects of indoor plants in the built healthcare environment: The mediating role of perceived attractiveness. *Preventive Medicine, 47*(3), 279–283.

Dogrusoy, I. T., & Tureyen, M. (2007). A field study on determination of preferences for windows in office environments. *Building and Environment, 42*(10), 3660–3668.

Dravigne, A., Waliczek, T. M., Lineberger, R. D., & Zajicek, J. M. (2008). The effect of live plants and window views of green spaces on employee perceptions of job satisfaction. *HortScience, 43*(1), 183–187.

Eldaly, K., Zaki, N., & El-Gizawi, L. (2016). The associations between daylight sufficiency in hospital wards and patient satisfaction with mental healthcare services: An egyptian sample. *Acta Medica International, 3*(2), 101–111.

Farley, K. M., & Veitch, J. A. (2001, August 15). *A room with a view: A review of the effects of windows on work and well-being*. Institute for Research in Construction, National Research Council Canada.

Galasiu, A. D., & Veitch, J. A. (2006). Occupant preferences and satisfaction with the luminous environment and control systems in daylit offices: A literature review. *Energy and Buildings, 38*(7), 728–742.

Glerup, H., Mikkelsen, K., Poulsen, L., Hass, E., Overbeck, S., Thomsen, J., Charles, P., & Eriksen, E. F. (2000). Commonly recommended daily intake of vitamin D is not sufficient if sunlight exposure is limited. *Journal of Internal Medicine, 247*(2), 260–268.

Haans, A. (2014). The natural preference in people's appraisal of light. *Journal of Environmental Psychology, 39*, 51–61.

Heerwagen, J. H., & Orians, G. H. (1986). Adaptations to windowlessness: A study of the use of visual decor in windowed and windowless offices. *Environment and Behavior, 18*(5), 623–639.

Higgins, D. M., Wischmeyer, P. E., Queensland, K. M., Sillau, S. H., Sufit, A. J., & Heyland, D. K. (2012). Relationship of vitamin D deficiency to clinical outcomes in critically ill patients. *Journal of Parenteral and Enteral Nutrition, 36*(6), 713–720.

Hofmann, P. B. (2018). Stress among healthcare professionals calls out for attention. *Journal of Healthcare Management, 63*(5), 294–297.

Jiang, S. (2015). Encouraging engagement with therapeutic landscapes: Using transparent spaces to optimize stress reduction in urban health facilities. *All Dissertations.* 1495. https://tigerprints.clemson.edu/all_dissertations/1495

Jiang, S., Powers, M., Allison, D., & Vincent, E. (2017). Informing healthcare waiting area design using transparency attributes: A comparative preference study. *HERD: Health Environments Research & Design Journal, 10*(4), 49–63.

Joarder, A., Price, A., & Mourshed, M. (2009, April 1). Systematic study of the therapeutic impact of daylight associated with clinical recovery. In M. Kagioglou, J. Barlow, A. Price, D. F. Gray, & C. Gray (Eds.), *Proceedings of PhD workshop of HaCIRIC's international conference 2009: Improving healthcare infrastructures through innovation* (pp. 25–31). Brighton, UK.

Kaplan, R. (2001). The nature of the view from home: Psychological benefits. *Environment and Behavior, 33*(4), 507–542.

Kaplan, R. (1993). The role of nature in the context of the workplace. *Landscape and Urban Planning, 26*(1–4), 193–201.

Kaplan, S., & Wendt, J. S. (1972). Preference and the visual environment: Complexity and some alternatives. *Environmental Design: Research and Practice, 6*, 75–76.

Kearney, A. R. (2006). Residential development patterns and neighborhood satisfaction: Impacts of density and nearby nature. *Environment and Behavior, 38*(1), 112–139.

Keep, P., James, J., & Inman, M. (1980). Windows in the intensive therapy unit. *Anaesthesia, 35*(3), 257–262.

Keep, P. J. (1977). Stimulus deprivation in windowless rooms. *Anaesthesia, 32*(7), 598–602.

Keighley, E. C. (1973). Visual requirements and reduced fenestration in offices—A study of multiple apertures and window area. *Building Science , 8*(4), 321–331.

Klepeis, N. E., Nelson, W. C., Ott, W. R., Robinson, J. P., Tsang, A. M., Switzer, P., Behar, J. V., Hern, S. C., & Engelmann, W. H. (2001). The National Human Activity Pattern Survey (NHAPS): A resource for assessing exposure to environmental pollutants. *Journal of Exposure Science & Environmental Epidemiology, 11*(3), 231–252.

Ko, W. H., Schiavon, S., Zhang, H., Graham, L. T., Brager, G., Mauss, I., & Lin, Y. W. (2020). The impact of a view from a window on thermal comfort, emotion, and cognitive performance. *Building and Environment, 175*, 106779.

Küller, R., & Lindsten, C. (1992). Health and behavior of children in classrooms with and without windows. *Journal of Environmental Psychology, 12*(4), 305–317.

Küller, R., & Wetterberg, L. (1996). The subterranean work environment: Impact on well-being and health. *Environment International, 22*(1), 33–52.

Kuo, F. E., & Sullivan, W. C. (2001). Environment and crime in the inner city: Does vegetation reduce crime?. *Environment and Behavior, 33*(3), 343–367.

Lankston, L., Cusack, P., Fremantle, C., & Isles, C. (2010). Visual art in hospitals: Case studies and review of the evidence. *Journal of the Royal Society of Medicine, 103*(12), 490–499.

Laurentin, C., Berrutto, V., Fontoynont, M., & Girault, P. (1998) Manual control of artificial lighting in a daylit space. In *3rd international conference on indoor air quality, ventilation and energy conservation in buildings* (pp. 175–180). Lyon, France.

Leather, P., Pyrgas, M., Beale, D., & Lawrence, C. (1998). Windows in the workplace: Sunlight, view, and occupational stress. *Environment and Behavior, 30*(6), 739–762.

Lottrup, L., Stigsdotter, U. K., Meilby, H., & Corazon, S. S. (2012). Associations between use, activities and characteristics of the outdoor environment at workplaces. *Urban Forestry & Urban Greening, 11*(2), 159–168.

Markus, T. A. (1967). The function of windows—A reappraisal. *Building Science, 2*(2), 97–121.

Mourshed, M., & Zhao, Y. (2012). Healthcare providers' perception of design factors related to physical environments in hospitals. *Journal of Environmental Psychology, 32*(4), 362–370.

Nagy, E., Yasunaga, S., & Kose, S. (1995). Japanese office employees' psychological reactions to their underground and above-ground offices. *Journal of Environmental Psychology, 15*(2), 123–134.

Najimi, A., Goudarzi, A. M., & Sharifirad, G. (2012). Causes of job stress in nurses: A cross-sectional study. *Iranian Journal of Nursing and Midwifery Research, 17*(4), 301–305

Nanda, U., Eisen, S., Zadeh, R. S., & Owen, D. (2011). Effect of visual art on patient anxiety and agitation in a mental health facility and implications for the business case. *Journal of Psychiatric and Mental Health Nursing, 18*(5), 386–393.

Ne'Eman, E., & Hopkinson, R. G. (1970). Critical minimum acceptable window size: A study of window design and provision of a view. *Lighting Research & Technology*, *2*(1), 17–27.

O'Dowd, E., O'Connor, P., Lydon, S., Mongan, O., Connolly, F., Diskin, C., McLoughlin, A., Rabbitt, L., McVicker, L., Reid-McDermott, B., & Byrne, D. (2018). Stress, coping, and psychological resilience among physicians. *BMC Health Services Research*, *18*(1), 1–11.

Omran, M. A. (2000). Analysis of solar radiation over Egypt. *Theoretical and Applied Climatology*, *67*(3), 225–240.

Oren, D. A., Wisner, K. L., Spinelli, M., Epperson, C. N., Peindl, K. S., Terman, J. S., & Terman, M. (2002). An open trial of morning light therapy for treatment of antepartum depression. *American Journal of Psychiatry*, *159*(4), 666–669.

Park, M. Y., Chai, C. G., Lee, H. K., Moon, H., & Noh, J. S. (2018). The effects of natural daylight on length of hospital stay. *Environmental Health Insights, 12.* https://doi.org/10.1177/1178630218812817

Park, S. H., & Mattson, R. H. (2009). Ornamental indoor plants in hospital rooms enhanced health outcomes of patients recovering from surgery. *The Journal of Alternative and Complementary Medicine*, *15*(9), 975–980.

Pati, D., Harvey, T. E. Jr., & Barach, P. (2008). Relationships between exterior views and nurse stress: An exploratory examination. *Health Environments Research & Design Journal*, *1*(2), 27–38.

Raanaas, R. K., Patil, G. G., & Hartig, T. (2012). Health benefits of a view of nature through the window: A quasi-experimental study of patients in a residential rehabilitation center. *Clinical Rehabilitation*, *26*(1), 21–32.

Rechel, B., Buchan, J., & McKee, M. (2009). The impact of health facilities on healthcare workers' well-being and performance. *International Journal of Nursing Studies*, *46*(7), 1025–1034.

Shepley, M. M., Gerbi, R. P., Watson, A. E., Imgrund, S., & Sagha-Zadeh, R. (2012). The impact of daylight and views on ICU patients and staff. *HERD: Health Environments Research & Design Journal*, *5*(2), 46–60.

Shikder, S. H., Mourshed, M., & Price, A. D. (2010). Optimisation of a daylight-window: Hospital patient room as a test case. In W. Tizani (Ed.), *Proceedings of the international conference on computing in civil and building engineering.* Nottingham University Press. http://orca.cf.ac.uk/51402/1/pf194.pdf

Sop Shin, W. (2007). The influence of forest view through a window on job satisfaction and job stress. *Scandinavian Journal of Forest Research*, *22*(3), 248–253.

Stimpfel, A. W., Sloane, D. M., & Aiken, L. H. (2012). The longer the shifts for hospital nurses, the higher the levels of burnout and patient dissatisfaction. *Health Affairs*, *31*(11), 2501–2509.

Stone, N. J. (1998). Windows and environmental cues on performance and mood. *Environment and Behavior*, *30*(3), 306–321.

Stone, N. J., & Irvine, J. M. (1994). Direct or indirect window access, task type, and performance. *Journal of Environmental Psychology*, *14*(1), 57–63.

Taylor, A. F., Kuo, F. E., & Sullivan, W. C. (2002). Views of nature and self-discipline: Evidence from inner city children. *Journal of Environmental Psychology*, *22*(1–2), 49–63.

Ulrich, R. S. (1984). View through a window may influence recovery from surgery. *Science*, *224*(4647), 420–421.

Veitch, J. A., Geerts, J., Charles, K. E., Newsham, G. R., & Marquardt, C. J. G. (2005). Satisfaction with lighting in open-plan offices: COPE field findings. *Proceedings of Lux Europa, 2005*, 414–417.

Veitch, J. A., Hine, D. W., & Gifford, R. (1993). End users' knowledge, beliefs, and preferences for lighting. *Journal of Interior Design, 19*(2), 15–26.

Verderber, S. (1986). Dimensions of person–window transactions in the hospital environment. *Environment and Behavior, 18*(4), 450–466.

Verderber, S., & Reuman, D. (1987). Windows, views, and health status in hospital therapeutic environments. *Journal of Architectural and Planning Research, 4*(2), 120–133.

Vinall, P. E. (1997). Design technology: What you need to know about circadian rhythms in healthcare design. *Journal of Healthcare Design, 9*, 141–144.

Vincent, E., Battisto, D., & Grimes, L. (2010a). The effects of presence and influence in nature images in a simulated hospital patient room. *HERD: Health Environments Research & Design Journal, 3*(3), 56–69.

Vincent, E., Battisto, D., Grimes, L., & McCubbin, J. (2010b). The effects of nature images on pain in a simulated hospital patient room. *HERD: Health Environments Research & Design Journal, 3*(3), 42–55.

Wells, B. W. P. (1965). Subjective responses to the lighting installation in a modern office building and their design implications. *Building Science, 1*(1), 57–68.

Wilson, L. M. (1972). Intensive care delirium: The effect of outside deprivation in a windowless unit. *Archives of Internal Medicine, 130*(2), 225–226.

World Health Organization. (1946). *Preamble to the Constitution of WHO as adopted by the International Health Conference, New York, 19 June–22 July 1946. The first ten years of the World Health Organization.* Author.

Wunsch, H., Gershengorn, H., Mayer, S. A., & Claassen, J. (2011). The effect of window rooms on critically ill patients with subarachnoid hemorrhage admitted to intensive care. *Critical Care, 15*(2), 1–10.

Zadeh, R. S., Shepley, M. M., Williams, G., & Chung, S. S. E. (2014). The impact of windows and daylight on acute-care nurses' physiological, psychological, and behavioral health. *HERD: Health Environments Research & Design Journal, 7*(4), 35–61.

4 Hospital Greenspaces and Some Usage Issues

Although integrating some sort of nature in a hospital is not a new concept, the previous inclusion of window views and greenspaces in hospitals was not carefully considered for therapeutic purposes. This chapter first reviews the people–nature relationships in hospitals in representative historical periods of European societies, with two waves of nature integration in hospital environments emphasized: the pavilion hospital plans advocated by Florence Nightingale in the mid-19th century and the tuberculosis sanatorium movement and its impacts on modern hospital design between the two world wars. Hospital greenspaces experienced a sharp decline, even fully disappearing in postwar modernist hospitals, until their revival in contemporary designs accompanying the shift to patient-centered care and evidence-based design. Although hospital greenspaces have become increasingly common in contemporary hospitals, some usage issues remain. Finally, this chapter documents two recent post-occupancy evaluation (POE) studies on a series of hospital greenspaces to conclude that the locations and spatial relationships between greenspaces and hospital interiors matter the usage patterns of those spaces.

People–Nature Relationship in Hospitals in History

A General Negligence

Growing evidence suggests the therapeutic effects of nature, and contemporary research has demonstrated such effects of greenspaces in hospitals on patient and staff outcomes. From the functional purposes of courtyards and orchards (for cultivating medicinal herbs and food and serving as cemeteries) in medieval cloisters to the catholic hospitals that followed the architectural traditions of arcades and interior courtyards, greenspaces have long been incorporated into hospital environments (Gerlach-Spriggs et al., 1998). However, early hospitals were based on "derived" plans rather than "designed plans," meaning that the configuration and exterior of the hospital were copied or synthesized from other building types without being purposefully designed for the function of nursing and healthcare

DOI: 10.4324/9781003122180-4

(Thompson & Goldin, 1975; Verderber & Fine, 2000). Therefore, the people–nature relationship within these first hospitals was incidental rather than meaningful. For example, the majority of the catholic hospitals of the Renaissance and Reformation Europe adapted plans from palaces or churches that walled their patients off from the outside; the windows in the patient wards were so high up on the wall that neither patients nor nurses could see the sun or gardens outside (Gerlach-Spriggs et al., 1998). Some asylums and hospitals shared a group value that individual buildings sometimes belonged within a designed landscape in which the ensemble was of greater importance than the individual buildings. As a result, the grand landscapes and formal gardens surrounding the hospitals were intended more for decorative than therapeutic purposes (Historic England, 2017). For example, the design of Bethlehem Hospital in Moorfields, London adopted a two-dimensional stage set with the front façade facing a grand open field. The open field was beneficial to the hospital in providing an airy context and uninterrupted views of the palace-like fronts. However, the backside of the Bethlehem hospital was plain and cramped, forming a striking contrast to its articulated openness in the front. An ancient Roman structure of London Wall, which was only 9 feet way, ran parallel to the rear façade of the hospital that prohibited any contact with the outside. It was almost impossible for patients to see the outside from those narrow, distanced windows, and the only accessible outdoor spaces were the two small exercise yards on either end of the narrow plan that were shielded from public view (Arnold, 2013).

From Courtyard Hospitals to Pavilion Plans

The general voluntary hospitals that emerged around the 18th century in England tended to arrange the hospital functions in the formats of building blocks around quadrangles, similar to those of an Oxford college—namely, the courtyard plans (Thompson & Goldin, 1975). Despite an embracing gesture between the architectural and landscape components, the patient beds in the building interiors were quite isolated in curtained cubicles as subdivided from a large hall, with the outside nature or views oriented back upon the patients. Mental health patients were then miserably placed in the cells in the basement. Post-1840 hospitals in England represented the earliest designed plans for hospitals, such as the pavilion hospitals and the nightingale wards, whose impacts lasted until the early 20th century (Thompson & Goldin, 1975). Landscaped grounds and small gardens in provincial hospitals emerging around this era served for four major functions: to provide fresh air; to allow opportunities for exercise; to be used as a kitchen garden; and as a place where the apothecary could grow medicinal plants. The front gardens of many hospitals were then evidently designed as ornamental grounds to be seen by people passing by (Hickman, 2013).

During the 19th century, the prevailing miasma theory impacted hospital design by emphasizing natural daylight and ventilation in hospital environments, which led to the emergence of the pavilion plans. The pavilion plans consisted of single- or double-story ward blocks, placed at right angles to a linking corridor oriented straight or enclosing a large central square; the pavilions were widely separated, usually by lawns or gardens. In the wards, complete cross-ventilation was achieved by opposite rows of tall, narrow, floor-to-ceiling windows (King, 1966). Windows in the pavilion hospitals were then purposefully designed to capture daylight and circulate fresh air, where a more relevant relationship was initiated between patients and the outside nature. According to Verderber's (Verderber, 2003; Verderber & Fine, 2000) summarization of the six waves of hospital architecture in history, the pavilion plan and nightingale wards in particular should be considered as the first truly modernist hospital planning efforts. Florence Nightingale, the founder of modern nursing and a miasmatists, advocated for the pavilion structures in her *Notes on Hospitals* (1863) and emphasized the importance of connecting patients with nature in her other book *Notes on Nursing: What It Is and What It Is Not* (1860). To receive sunlight at all hours of the day, patient ward should be as nearly as possible north-south oriented, and the windows should take up one-third of the wall space (Thompson & Goldin, 1975). There should be at least one window to every two beds; rows of tall windows should be placed on walls facing the wards to encourage good ventilation, and beds should be arranged adjacent to the windows where direct access to a window and natural daylight from a patient's bedside is possible. Nightingale suggested that hospitals "must be as like a home and as unlike a hospital as possible" (1863, p. 108). In her notes, she wrote:

> I have seen, in fevers, (and felt, when I was a fever patient myself,) the most acute suffering produced from the patient (in a hut) not being able to see out of window, and the knots in the wood being the only view. I shall never forget the rapture of fever patients over a bunch of bright-colored flowers. I remember (in my own case) a nosegay of wild flowers being sent me, and from that moment recovery becoming more rapid. People say the effect is only on the mind. It is no such thing. The effect is on the body, too. Little as we know about the way in which we are affected by form, by color, and light, we do know this, that they have an actual physical effect. (Nightingale, 1860, p. 45)

Using a series of figure-ground diagrams, Figure 4.1 demonstrates the prevailing building layouts of older hospitals in representative historic periods. Despite the inclusion of courtyards and greenspaces in some layouts, the people–nature interactions in older hospitals were vague and negligent. The design of mental asylums combined buildings and gardens as part of the care regime; doctors believed that contact with nature could

The Monastery of Cluny,
France (about 1157)
The Medieval

Hospital of St. Louis,
Paris (1608)
Forerunner of the pavilion plan

Bethlehem Hospital,
London (1676)
The Renaissance palace hospital

Guy's Hospital for Incurables,
London (1725)
The courtyard plan

Pennsylvania Hospital,
Philadelphia (1755)
The Kirkbride plan

St. Thomas's Hospital,
London (1871)
The pavilion hospital - Nightingale ward

Buildings
Grounds

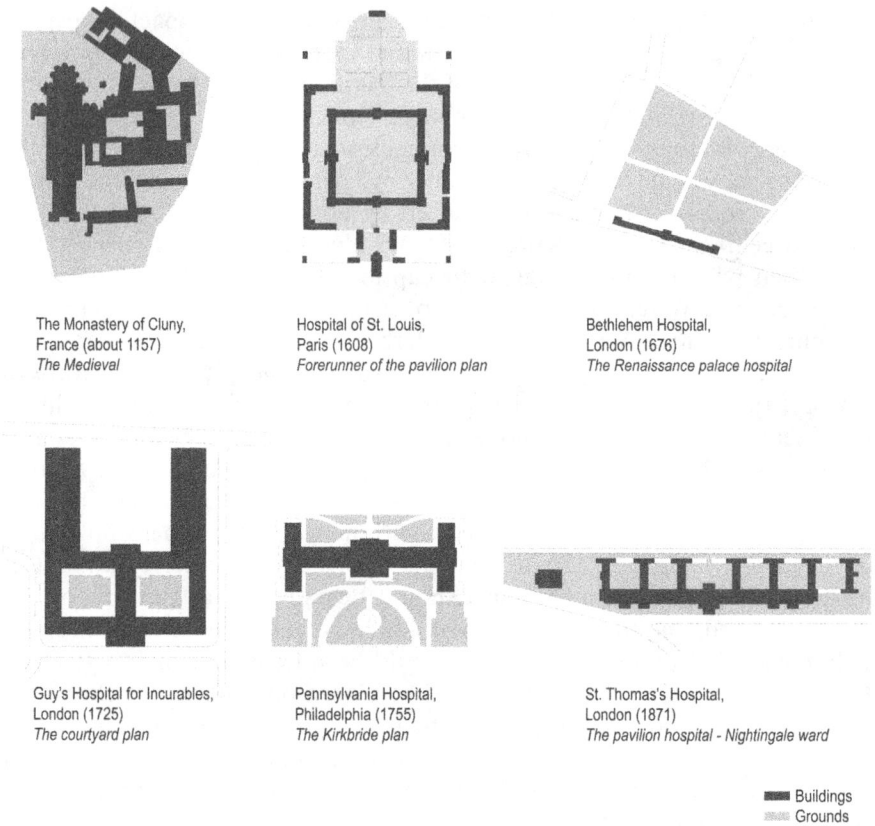

Figure 4.1 Figure-ground diagrams of building layouts for the representative hospitals in history

Source: Drawn by Shan Jiang and Udday Datta

improve patients' health and correctly organized buildings could augment
or diminish such contact (Theodore, 2017). The Kirkbride plan, a design
template for early psychiatric institutes in the United States advocated by
American psychiatrist Thomas Story Kirkbride in the mid-19th century,
was created based on the idea that controlled nature was essential to heal
the disturbed mind (Tomes, 1994). As summarized by Cooper Marcus and
Sachs (2014, p. 9), the Kirkbride plan suggested that asylums should be
located in the countryside no less than two miles from a large city. The
facility should occupy at least 100 acres of land or half an acre per patient,
of which at least 50 acres should be dedicated to gardens and landscaped
grounds. Patient wards for "the most excited class" of patients should have
large windows and pleasant views.

People–nature engagement in hospitals was shortly ascendant in the mid-
19th-century pavilion hospitals and asylums, in which large windows were

designed to look at greenspaces between patient wards. Once it was determined that germs are the carrier of contagious diseases but not miasma, and antiseptics and basic hygiene could prevent the spread of germs, physical separation in the pavilion or courtyard hospitals became unnecessary. The role of the general hospital changed along with the rise of surgery and scientific medicine in early 20th century. Hospitals shifted the focus to acute care, and patients' length of stay was significantly shortened due to separating the convalescence function from the original healthcare system (Hickman, 2013). Hospital greenspaces declined, and the window views to the outside were not prioritized for patients' needs until the movement of modernist architecture alongside the tuberculosis pandemic in the early 20th century.

Lessons Learned from Tuberculosis Sanatoriums

Tuberculosis Sanatorium Movement

The tuberculosis pandemic from the middle of the 19th century to the middle of the 20th century in Europe and North America led to social movements, legislations, and waves of sanatorium construction. In 1882, the discovery of the germ theory revealed that tuberculosis was not genetic but contagious; isolation was key to prevent the spread of tuberculosis, and before the widespread usage of antibiotics in the 1950s the effective relief of the disease relied on good hygiene, balanced nutrition, gentle exercise, and a regime of fresh air and sunbaths (Grahn, 2015; Martini et al., 2018). The therapeutic properties of ultraviolet light were believed effective in destroying the tubercle bacilli; therefore, sunbaths, also known as heliotherapy, became a necessary feature in every tuberculosis facility at the time. The standard of care for tuberculosis was primarily environmental. Patients could stay in single rooms or rooms with a few beds, which usually provided window views onto large terraces where patients could receive the sunlight treatment. The buildings were surrounded by spacious meadows or tree-lined landscapes, where guests could go for long healthy walks (Martini et al., 2018; Warren, 2006). The founding structures of sanitoriums in the United States were established by Dr. Edward Livingston Trudeau around the Saranac Lake region in New York between 1873 and 1945. The Saranac Lake model adopted a specific building type, known as "cure cottages," in which patients stayed in smaller groups with balanced isolation and socialization. To maximize patients' exposure to fresh air and sunlight, the oversized windows and sliding glass were added around the decks of the cottage-style buildings; patients spent at least eight hours a day resting on these "curing porches" and looking at the amplified nature views (Gallos, 1985).

It has been well documented that the tuberculosis sanatorium movement impacted modernism in architecture (Theodore, 2017). The modernist features of buildings, such as flat roofs, balconies and terraces, white-painted concrete structures, and the generous use of glass and windows, have coincided with the needs of fresh air, sunlight, hygiene, and dignity for the social housing since the late 19th century in Europe (Campbell, 2005; Hobday, 1997). Reuben Rainey, a professor emeritus of landscape architecture at the University of Virginia, commented that the landscape as a healing element was very important to the modernist architecture as the whole idea was to bring the outdoors indoors.

> Modernist architects such as Richard Neutra and Le Corbusier were very concerned with the therapeutic benefits of siting their buildings in nature. Neutra's highly transparent houses allowed the landscape to flow seamlessly into the interior and Le Corbusier often sited his buildings in pastoral landscapes that have been proven to be highly effective in relieving stress.[1]

The flat roofs and terraces in Le Corbusier's designs were believed to be the result of having seen some early tuberculosis sanatoriums in Switzerland (Campbell, 2005). Le Corbusier (1931/1985) considered the possibilities of holistic health while living in a city environment and suggested that flats each have their own garden terrace while a kilometer-long running track be included on the roof of the apartment block to enable residents to run in the fresh air.

In the book *Light, Air and Openness*, art historian Paul Overy (2007) explored the preoccupation with cleanliness, health, hygiene, sunlight, fresh air, and openness as representative characteristics of modern architecture between the two world wars. The Zonnestraal Sanatorium near Hilversum, the Netherlands, originally built in 1925–1931 and restored in about 2010, was considered a masterpiece of the early 20th-century modernist building (Figure 4.2). Impacted by the De Stijl esthetics, Zonnestraal denoted "a spiritual freeing of the structure from any obvious weight" (Campbell, 2005, p. 470). As implicated by the name of the facility—*Zonnestraal* meaning sunbeam—the oversized windows immersed the building in the pine woods surrounding the original site, the white-painted concrete walls with the "enormous swathes of glass creating an almost unbelievable intensity of light which would have given patients and staff a sense of continual emotional and spiritual uplift" (Overy, 2007, p. 8).

Paimio Sanatorium

The Site

The construction method and layout for the Zonnestraal Sanatorium greatly impressed Alvar Aalto and influenced his design of the Paimio Sanatorium in Finland (1929–1933), where the personal needs of patients and staff were emphasized (Campbell, 2005). Paimio Sanatorium was placed in a pine-wood forest in Paimio in southwest Finland. The overall site arrangement

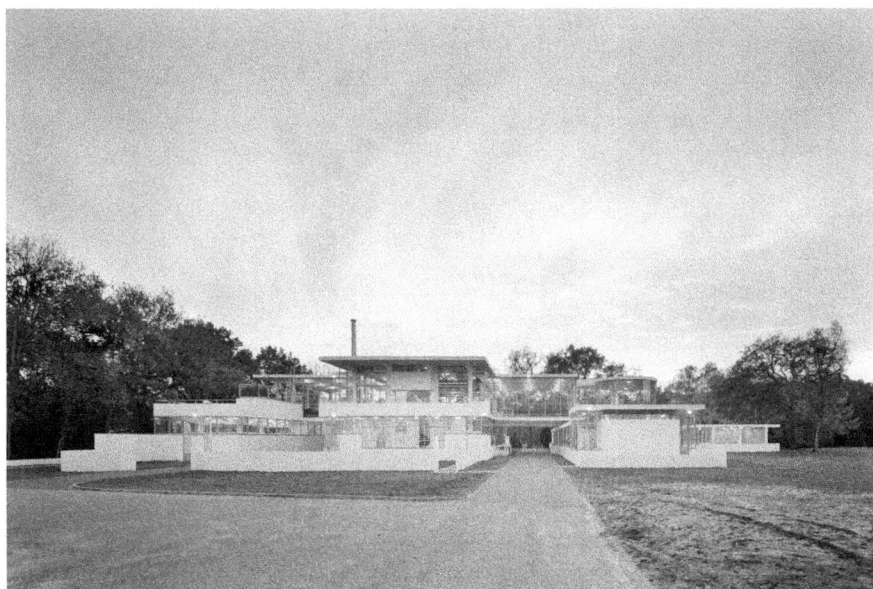

Figure 4.2 The main building of Zonnestraal Sanatorium, originally designed by architect Jan Duiker in 1926, and restored by Bierman Henket architecten and Wessel de Jonge architecten in 2003

Source: © Michel Kievits/Sybolt Voeten

was intended to minimize the spread of disease and disruption to patients and optimize natural daylight and ventilation through unique orientation and fenestration (20th Century Architecture, n.d.). The main building—a seven-story patient wing accommodating 145 rooms—was carefully oriented as a light trap to catch all the available sunlight (Overy, 2007). The institutional functions were deconstructed into different building wings arranged asymmetrically while simultaneously being based on a controlled system of coordinates. According to Heikinheimo's (2016, 2018a, 2018b) analyses and the documentation of the Paimio Sanatorium Conservation Management Plan (Heikkonen, 2016), the patients' wing (A) adopted a long, narrow footprint, where the patient rooms were arranged along a 100-foot single-loaded corridor. The sun balconies joined the A-wing at a 20° angle, running parallel to the B-wing that houses supportive functions including reception, operating theatre, treatment, dining, library, and workshops. The circulation area connecting the A and B wings was at right angles in relation to the A wing, while the C-wing (kitchen and laundry) joined the B wing at a 45° angle. The sun balconies and the dining and work halls in the B wing faced directly south; the halls were higher on the south than on the north side, which ensured that the sunlight could penetrate into the northern corners of the space (see Figure 4.3).

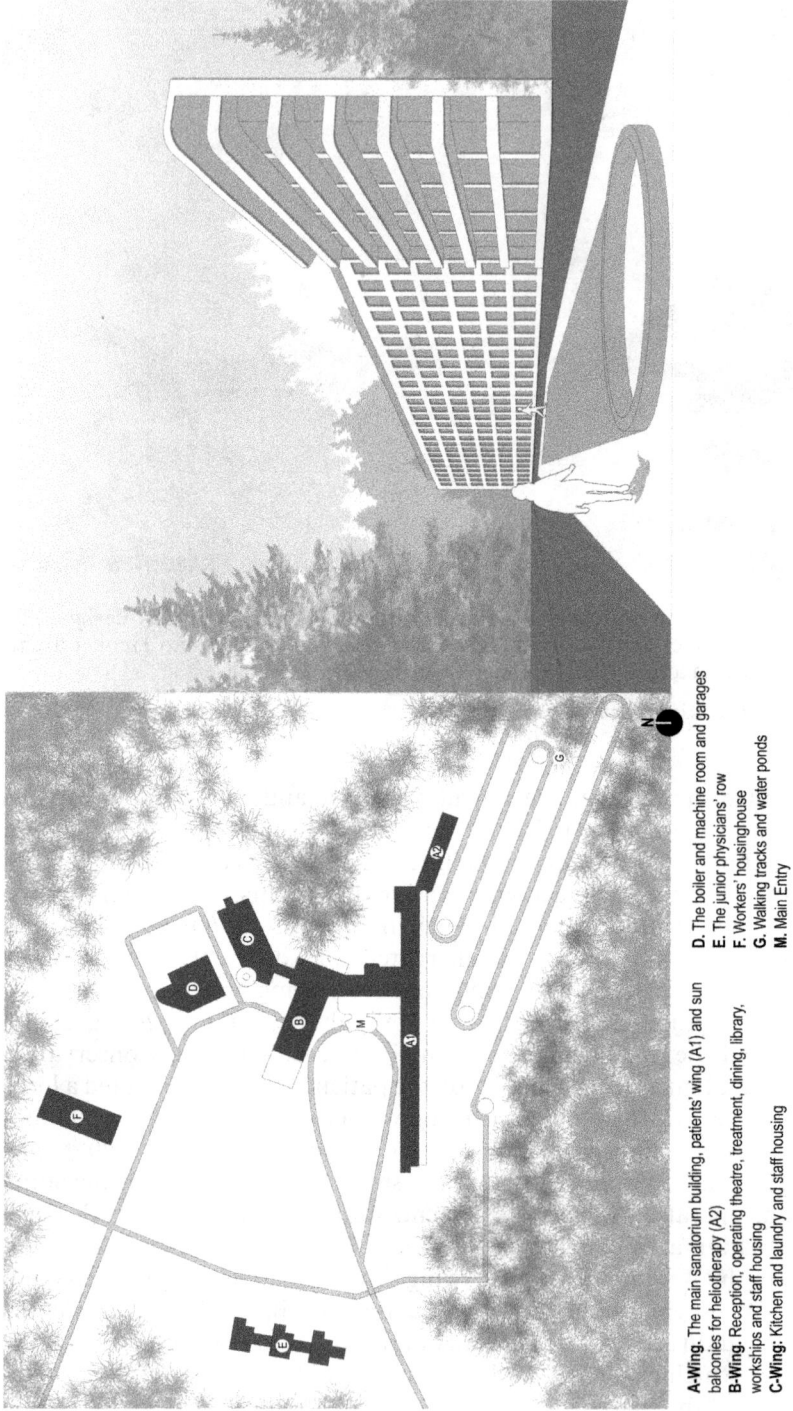

A-Wing. The main sanatorium building, patients' wing (A1) and sun balconies for heliotherapy (A2)
B-Wing. Reception, operating theatre, treatment, dining, library, workships and staff housing
C-Wing: Kitchen and laundry and staff housing

D. The boiler and machine room and garages
E. The junior physicians' row
F. Workers' housinghouse
G. Walking tracks and water ponds
M. Main Entry

Figure 4.3 Paimio Sanatorium site plan (left) and the view of the sun balconies for heliotherapy from the walking track (right)

Source: Drawn by Shan Jiang and Udday Datta

The Windows

Windows were thoughtfully considered in the design of the Paimio Sanatorium. The windows of the patients' ward faced south–southeast toward the morning sun. Informed by medical experts' opinions and patients' needs in both sunlight and shade, Aalto fixed wooden Venetian blinds outside the patient windows to regulate the lighting and added canvas sun awnings to the south-facing windows in the B wing. Considering the expense of using all-steel windows in an era of financial depression in Finland, Aalto invented a new type of hybrid window (wooden frames with the use of steel T-profiles for structural support) that expanded horizontally to allow for continuous ventilation even in winter seasons. This new window was known as the "health window":

> The patient room has the following characteristics, among others: morning sun on the patients' beds; afternoon sun on the front part of the room, in front of the window. Double-glazed windows in wood with L-shaped frames, with permanent ventilation through glass panes with vertical openings. Exposure to the sun can be adjusted using external blinds .... (Aalto, 1932, p. 80, quoted in Heikinheimo, 2018b, p. 5)

Aalto eventually compromised the L-shaped windows and leveled the bottom parts for hygiene reasons, but he creatively changed the shape of the floor so that it curved up near the window, making the window appear to reach the floor. A layer of windows ran along the corridor in the opposite direction of the patient rooms; the window height was intentionally increased to be the same height as the patient room door so that another layer of window views would be introduced to the patients when keeping the door open.

The Indoor–Outdoor Transition

The indoor–outdoor transition is another salient feature at the Paimio Sanatorium. Between the wings of the main building, a number of different courtyards and gardens were built. Three building wings enclosed the main entrance and a loop of the pathway, forming a landscaped courtyard; generous window views of this central courtyard can be easily seen from the entrance hall, stair landings, dining room, library, and main corridor in the patient wing. According to Heikinheimo's (2018a) interpretation, Aalto believed in the importance of socialization in a hospital environment, including that it was important to see and to be seen. The sanatorium entrance was like the steps up to a 19th-century theatre: a social stage (Heikinheimo, 2018a). To the east end of the patient wing, each level of patient rooms has a dedicated sun terrace. On the top floor of the patient wing, a spacious sun deck with mountain pines planted in containers was designed to accommodate up to 120 patients to receive heliotherapy while inhaling the scent of the surrounding pinewoods—an early form of aromatherapy (Overy, 2007). Looking down from the sun deck, five circular ponds were built in the original plan, bordered by landscaped paths that were arranged in parallel to the direction of the sun deck. Patients, visitors, and medical staff members could walk along the footpaths for mild exercise or full immersion in the pinewood forest.

Despite the later criticism of modern hospitals as healing machines, particularly those designed following Rationalism and the International Style (Verderber & Fine, 2000), a few tuberculosis sanatoriums' architecture in the early stage of modernism sparked the romanticization and humanization of machine architecture (Kim, 2009). As advocated by Aalto, patient populations' special needs should be addressed in environmental design; technical functionalism in modern hospitals is correct only if enlarged to cover the psychological and psychophysical field (Aalto, 1940/1997).

Greenspaces in Contemporary Hospitals

The Revival of Hospital Greenspaces

Greenspaces and people–nature engagement in hospital environments experienced two evident waves of ascendants in the recent history: one in the mid to late 19th century, when pavilion plans and Nightingale wards were prevalent, and another echoing the tuberculosis sanatorium movement between the two world wars. The International Style dominated hospital design in the United States and Europe for at least 40 years after World War II; greenspaces declined and even completely disappeared in those tower hospitals (Strickland, 2017; Verderber & Fine, 2000). Many social, economic, and cultural factors caused hospital design to shift from an emphasis of medical *care* to *cure*. Hospitals arrived at the apex of pure functionalism driven by the machine-based medicine and technical quality of care, the demanding needs of medical efficacy and efficiency, the evolving requirements for medical training and education, legislation, and the suddenly declining amount of funding for medical care and hospital construction (Theodore, 2017; Verderber & Fine, 2000). According to Verderber and Fine (2000), humanists' criticism of modernist hospitals was based on several observations, where "form follows function" was interpreted in an overly restrictive way. Key decision makers tended to oversimplify the daily needs of the building occupants, and patients and staff members' needs were less prioritized than the machines housed within the hospital. In addition, general designers lacked specific knowledge of the myriad implications of the healthcare buildings for patients and the general public.

The current revival of hospital greenspaces arrived with the accompaniment of the rejection of modernism and the exploration of patient-centered environmental design since the late 20th century. Gerteis and colleagues'

(1993) seminal edition *Through the Patient's Eyes* set the grounds for a humanistic framework, namely patient-centered care, in the design and delivery of the healthcare system. Healthcare planning and design have gradually shifted the focus on evidence-based design and the design of a holistically supportive environment for all user groups—patients, healthcare providers and staff members, and families and visitors (Ulrich et al., 2004). Viewing nature through windows has been proven associated with improved health outcomes among patients and other user groups by accumulating research evidence, which will be elaborated in the next chapter. Newly emerged professions, such as occupational and physical therapy, and horticultural therapy, use gardening as a means of both physical and mental health rehabilitation. The Facility Guidelines Institute, the authoritative source for guidance on health and residential care facility planning, design, and construction in the United States, added "access to nature" to the Environment of Care section as a new key element since their 2014 Guidelines for Design and Construction of Hospitals and Outpatient Facilities, which officially remarks the important role of nature in the physical environment of healthcare facilities (Cooper Marcus & Sachs, 2013; Facility Guidelines Institute, 2014).

In the examination of the typologies, forms, and locations of greenspaces in contemporary hospitals, Cooper Marcus and Sachs (2014, pp. 36–46) classified 16 types of healing gardens in contemporary hospitals based on their field notes of hospital visits from 1995 to 2012 in North American and European countries:

• Extensive Landscape Grounds
• Borrowed Landscape
• Nature and Fitness Trials
• Landscaped Setback
• Front Porch
• Entry Garden
• Backyard Garden
• "Tucked Away" Garden
• Courtyard
• "Hole-in-a-Donut" Garden
• Plaza
• Roof Garden
• Roof Terrace
• Peripheral Garden
• Atrium Garden
• Viewing Garden

Contemporary hospitals intend to incorporate greenspaces in the site design; nonetheless, the people–nature relationship in many hospitals have still been insufficiently emphasized. Hospital greenspaces are usually considered as "what separates buildings or what's left over" or "a reserve for future expansion of the healthcare facility and [will] eventually be built over" (Cooper Marcus, 2007, p. 21). It has been overlooked that the spatial relationship between hospital interiors and the greenspaces on a medical campus influence people's usage pattern of the space. Maintaining a patient–centered perspective, Whitehouse and colleagues (2001) conducted a POE on the garden space of a pediatric hospital and found that garden use was accompanied by increased consumer satisfaction, enhanced emotional respite for visitors, and reduced pain and distress among patients. People who used the garden spaces appreciated the various therapeutic attributes; however, the garden was not as frequently or effectively utilized as planned due to the low visibility (Whitehouse et al., 2001). Sherman and colleagues' (2005) study found that the largest garden in a cancer center with the most direct patient access was the most used space. Pasha's (2013) study further revealed that a lack of knowledge about the existence of the garden, low visibility, and limited accessibility to the garden spaces were major barriers to garden visitation in a hospital environment.

Current Usage Issues of Hospital Greenspaces through Post-Occupancy Evaluations

Post-Occupancy Evaluation (POE)

A POE in architecture can be defined as "the process of evaluating buildings in a systematic and rigorous manner after they have been built and occupied for some time" from the perspective of occupants using the setting (Preiser et al., 1988, p. 3; Cooper Marcus & Francis, 1998). POE as a research strategy has been well established in the field of healthcare research and design, and there has been advocacy that hospital greenspaces, like what has been achieved with architecture and interiors, should take steps toward evaluation and certification through rigorous POEs (Cooper Marcus & Sachs, 2013). Prior scholars have employed the POE strategy to study hospital gardens and their impacts on various user groups, which has helped summarize effective suggestions for the design of future hospital greenspaces (Davis, 2011; Heath & Gifford, 2001; Sherman et al., 2005).

According to Cooper Marcus and Sachs (2014), the three most common types of POEs in hospital garden evaluations are indicative (i.e., a short walkthrough evaluation sometimes involving the use of an audit), investigative (i.e., prompted by issues identified during an indicative POE to cover those issues in more depth), and diagnostic; among which the diagnostic POE is the most comprehensive evaluation strategy and utilizes multiple methods. An ideal diagnostic POE should include the following components (Cooper Marcus & Sachs, 2014, pp. 309–310): project context and site analysis, interviews with the original designer, interviews with hospital staff members, observations of the maintenance situations, and examination of users' behaviors through behavior traces, behavior mapping, and interviews. Naomi Sachs (2017) advocates for diagnostic POEs that they should also include an audit of the elements that are (or should be) in the hospital greenspace. The Healthcare Garden Evaluation Toolkit (H-GET), a standardized toolkit, has been developed and proven effective in the evaluation of gardens in healthcare facilities. The H-GET recommends four components in a diagnostic POE of hospital greenspace: (1) audit the design elements using the Garden Assessment Tool for Evaluators (GATE); (2) staff and patient/visitor surveys; (3) behavior mapping; and (4) stakeholder interviews (Sachs, 2017).

Study Sites

Following the diagnostic POE protocol suggested by Cooper Marcus and Sachs (2014), Jiang and Kaljevic (2017a, 2017b) conducted two POE studies on two general hospitals in the United States, evaluating a total of 14 hospital greenspaces in detail regarding the landscape performance efficacy and usage patterns of the spaces. Two hospital sites were jointly selected by the research team and project funding agency[2] because of the exemplary design of the greenspaces on the two medical campuses. The two hospitals' landscape environments share several similarities: They were designed by the same firm and guided by similar design philosophies, both were built around the same time, and there are similar programs in many garden spaces. The major differences of the hospital greenspaces are the locations and spatial relationships between the gardens and buildings, and the visual and physical access by different user groups. The similarities of the two hospital greenspaces could help control and reduce distractive variables when making cross-case comparisons to explore how the locations influence the usability of the greenspaces (Table 4.1).

Findings from the Site Evaluation and Audit

A mixture of POE methods and instruments were employed in the study, including an archival analysis of the original design drawings and documents, an interview with the original landscape designer, the evaluation and audit of hospital greenspaces, observation and behavior mapping, and focus groups with stakeholder representatives (Jiang et al., 2018). A total of 14 greenspaces were evaluated, and six gardens from the two hospitals were selected for detailed evaluation and audit using the GATE tool. In general, all garden designs were strong in terms of planting considerations, esthetics, and maintenance, which helped provide pleasant views to various user groups from within the hospital. The Dining Patio (B-1) at Hospital B received the highest total GATE score (i.e., 8.8 out of 10), followed by the Dining Plaza and Commemorative Garden at Hospital A (A-1) (i.e., 8.7 out of 10). All garden designs could improve the variety and activities associated with pathways within spaces, such as spaces and

Table 4.1 Comparison of Greenspaces at Hospital A versus Hospital B

Comparison items	Hospital A	Hospital B
At-a-glance information		
Location and climate zone	Kentucky, Humid Subtropical	New Jersey, Humid Subtropical
Campus size and capacity	157 acres, 477 beds	127 acres, 368 beds
Impervious area	67% of the site	68% of the site
Retention/detention water area	8 retention ponds, total 15 acres of surface water	40 acres of reserved or newly constructed wetlands
Open to local communities	Yes, free parking and kids' playgrounds open to local communities	Parking is not free, but the landscape is accessible by local communities
Completion time	June 2013	May 2011
Hospital garden location and typology		
Extensive landscaped grounds	Yes, mainly flat	Yes, with extensive topographical changes
Nature and fitness trails	Yes, playgrounds along the trail system connecting to the community greenway	Yes, internal trails plus bike lanes
Entry garden	Yes, entrance of Medical Office Building (MOB)	Yes, entrance of Children's Emergency Department (ED)
Courtyard	Yes, central courtyard, memorial	Yes, main entrance courtyard
Plaza	Yes, behind the inpatient, dining, and memorial areas	Yes, near front entrance and dining area
Roof garden/terrace	Yes, one roof garden, no physical access, for viewing only	Yes, three roof gardens/terraces in total: two shared by the Neonatal Intensive Care Unit (NICU) and Pediatric Intensive Care Unit (PICU), with both physical and visual access, and one near the staff entrance on the roof of the cafeteria space with both physical and visual access
Viewing garden	Yes, in the staff lounge area without physical access	No purely viewing garden

features for therapists to work with patients, and provide more opportunities for users to experience the sense of "being away" through landscape designs. The lack of tables and water features as well as insufficient lighting, wayfinding, and amenities were found to contribute to lower GATE scores (Figures 4.4 and 4.5).

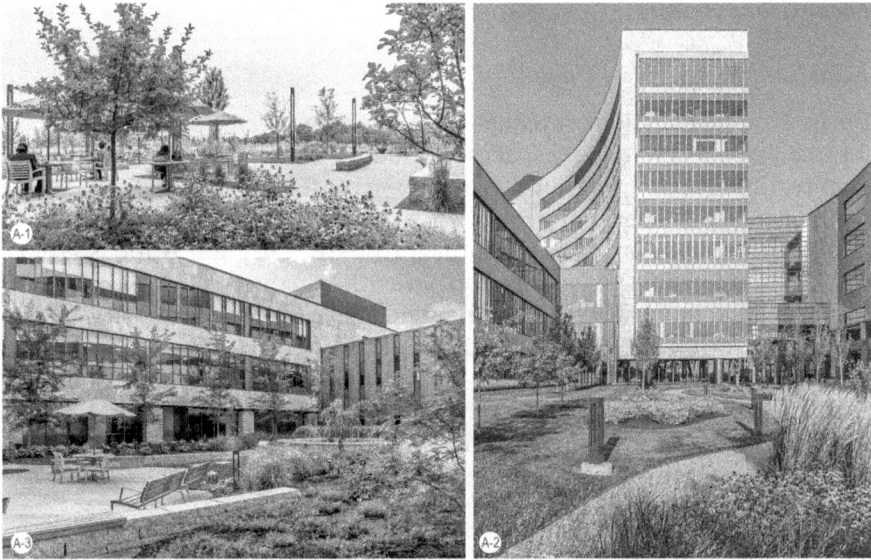

Figure 4.4 Hospital A Dining Plaza and Commemorative Garden (A-1), Entrance Rain Garden (A-2), and the Main Courtyard (A-3)

Source: © HGA Architects and Engineers. Research conducted as part of the Landscape Architecture Foundation's 2017 Case Study Investigation Program, materials used with permission

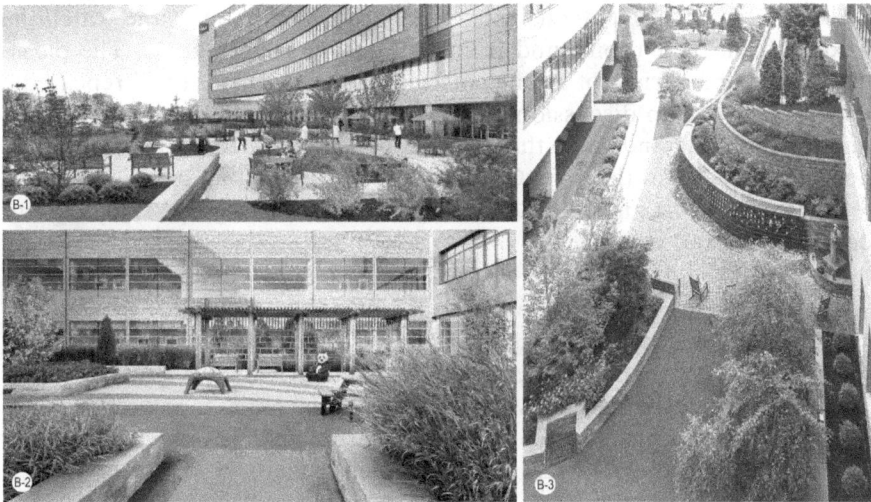

Figure 4.5 Hospital B Dining Patio (B-1), Children's ED Therapeutic Garden (B-2), and the Angel's Courtyard (B-3)

Source: © HGA Architects and Engineers. Research conducted as part of the Landscape Architecture Foundation's 2017 Case Study Investigation Program, materials used with permission

Focus Group Results

Visual and Experiential Quality

Focus group discussions revealed the prevailing themes of usage patterns for the two hospital greenspaces, including (1) visual and experiential quality, (2) wellness programs and supportive features, and (3) landscape maintenance and operation.

The most prevailing theme identified from the Hospital A focus groups was the extraordinary visual and experiential quality of the overall landscape design on campus. Therapeutic landscape environments helped increase staff job satisfaction, and all interviewed participants expressed a sense of pride working in this facility because of the appraisals they frequently receive from patients, families, and visitors. Hospital nurses described that having opportunities to temporarily get away and take a break in a garden space could help reduce their work-related stress and improve their mood status:

> It is the space to get away, peaceful, it is calming you know, it is beautiful... I think that helps definitely to recharge and go back to the situation where you were. And hopefully if you deal with patients, your situation is much easier, after you have that experience. (Nurse, Hospital A focus group)

Based on the staff members' observations and conversations with patients and family members, patients enjoy the extraordinary views and watch the wildlife from their rooms and from the outside seating areas. The pleasure of having a variety of animal species on site was mentioned repeatedly during focus group discussions at Hospital A. The conversations focused on bird-watching and geese that nested on campus, specifically around the pedestrian bridge at the Rain Garden (A-2) during mating season. Patients' feelings of comfort and peace often came from watching and enjoying outdoor scenery and wildlife:

> They feel private in this hospital and a sense of peace when they go outside and look out the windows, a sense of comfort for our patients. And I would say probably at least 90% of them have made comments about what they see from their window. Some of the patients ask to sit by the window so they can watch this whole drama playing out with the geese and the ducks.... (Nurse, Hospital A focus group).

Similar to the findings from Hospital A, the most prevailing topic in both focus group interviews at Hospital B was the visual accessibility of the greenspaces on campus from various indoor areas. For hospital staff, the 360-degree views from the hospital building offer many more benefits than the physical use of the various greenspaces outside. Such a conclusion is completely understandable considering that employees usually have only 30-minute lunch breaks per day, and the use of outdoor space is limited by season and weather conditions. When referring to the data collected through observational studies and behavior mapping at the Dining Patio (B-1), on average good weather days, the hospital staff members spend an average of 12 minutes outside during their lunch breaks. Having visual access to greenspaces could help reduce staff's stress during work, as stated by one nursing staff member:

> It makes you feel calm...and if you can just look out there sometimes, especially if is the stressful kind of message getting delivered. You see pretty flowers, or the fall foliage.... It is just kind of like we can do this! (Nurse, Hospital B focus group)

Wellness Programs and Supportive Features

A hierarchical trail system was established on both hospital sites forming an essential wellness program to support patients' rehabilitation and promote green exercise among staff members and local community residents. The medical team at Hospital A used different areas of the grounds for patients' rehabilitation activities, weather permitting, and the nursing staff was always open to new suggestions on how to improve and accelerate patients' recovery process by using the exterior areas. The trails provided opportunities for walking with different types of physical challenges, such as ramps, stairs, concrete, and gravel. According to care providers, patients need authentic outside conditions to recuperate and rebuild their confidence after an operation or injury. Furthermore, for disabled patients, the exterior of the hospital represents a safe environment and a neutral zone where they can work with their therapist and prepare for life outside the hospital:

> And once they cannot walk you are in the sense of pressure, you have community sidewalk, and if they are going to be in wheelchair they are going to have to use that. So that is an opportunity to practice in a safe environment with a therapist. It gives them the opportunity to gain confidence even the fact that they count on other people who are not patients, I think is good, because they—many times people, when they have a stroke, for some reason they feel embarrassed. (Nurse administrator, Hospital A focus group)

Staff members indicated that they usually use their break time to stretch their legs by walking along the trail in the Rain Garden, which is the closest to the hospital, because they have very limited break time. The ground maintenance employees confirmed that the trails near the building are the most frequently used based on their everyday observations. Many staff members found that having places that they can not only view from inside, but also in which they can sit and rest outside as well as use to improve their wellness was the most beneficial part of the campus design:

> I see a lot of the same staff members who walk on the farthest part of large walking trail, they sit on those benches by themselves, they would take their lunch break out, just quiet, and they walk back in. It is almost every day that the weather is good. (Staff member, Hospital A focus group)

> The wellness element that is not only for visitors, for patients that they can get out, but for employees too. I just love that peace of it; there is like pieces of exercise equipment, there are on some of the trails, and that to me is such a gift for employees. When I come up for meetings, I have been recharged. (Regular visitor, Hospital A focus group)

The community members also used the trails for different types of activities on an everyday basis, such as walking, biking, running, and walking with their children in strollers. The hospital provides parking spaces for local community members, and the campus will eventually be strategically linked to the local green belt project as part of a larger system of greenway. The longer trails that are further away from Hospital A's buildings are equipped with exercise equipment and seating. As interview participants commented, those trails would be used more by hospital residents if proper signage was added or if more people were educated of their existence. All interviewed participants stated that the wellness programs and design features on campus facilitate social bonding among local community members:

> I am on the ground out there so I see things...lots of people using the trail, on a schedule. So, there are lots of people that are living close here that come with the vehicle and park on the parking lot and they would come here every day and ride the bikes, walk the dogs, let the kids play on the playground.... (Maintenance staff member, Hospital B focus group)

Landscape Maintenance and Operation

Extensive landscaped grounds were present on both hospital sites. A great variety of flora, fauna, and wildlife species were thriving on the Hospital A site. Hospital A was designed to include approximately 85 acres of prairie and grassland habitat. The investigators identified vastly opposing attitudes about the wild appearances of native plants on certain parts of the site; some participants highly praised the native grassland and wildflowers and the overall sense of escape and peace those plant materials created on site whereas others preferred manicured lawns and a "golf course" type of appearance, resulting in different maintenance strategies contrary to the initial design intents in certain areas. The majority of the focus group participants stressed that the public needs to be educated about sustainable design with native planting materials. As one maintenance staff member commented:

> I am not sure everybody understands our grassland exterior. So, lots of times they think that they are just letting the grass become overgrown. And that is not the situation. So, I would know is there a way to, you know, like to put up the sign... I know you cannot just put all the details or something for somebody who drives by. But I hear that comment: Why are they letting the grass grow? That is not, it's not what is happened, because it is grassland area and you do not want anything to be there.... (Maintenance staff member, Hospital B focus group)

The landscape maintenance issues and usage conflicts were frequently discussed during the focus groups at Hospital B. The landscape maintenance staff expressed concerns about maintenance challenges associated with green roof plantings and water features, such as the water wall at the Angel's Courtyard (B-3). Unlike Hospital A, whose green roof was used as a viewing garden that only authorized staff could enter, Hospital B had a series of green terraces open to all users. The rooftop gardens were covered with planting trays, which are not resistant to intensive physical activities. Located at the pediatric units, young visitors or patients' siblings participating in activities on the lawn may cause damage to plants. The handrails that enclose the upper-level rooftop garden meet building standards, but curious young visitors tend to climb on the handrails and overlook lower levels of terraces, creating a considerable safety hazard. As a result, staff must limit these visitors' usage of the rooftop garden spaces.

Interviewees also expressed that having more color in designs, such as colorful plant species and bloomers in the planting palette or some colorful decorations on the walls for the winter season, could help attract more users and keep them outside longer:

> I also think we need some color because right now it's just the pergola and the seating, and it's all green. Like we need something to make it more welcoming because you go out there you see something in green for so long, and then it's like this is boring. (Nurse administrator, Hospital B focus group)

For safety and maintenance considerations, certain gardens were not operated according to the intent of the original design. For example, the design of the Angel's Courtyard (B-3) included several entrances along the perimeter of the garden, but visitors have been restricted from directly entering it from the interior. Therefore, users must walk a longer distance and enter the courtyard from outside. A lack of direct physical access creates a significant barrier to the use of some hospital greenspaces.

Garden Locations Matter

Results from multiple data sources revealed that having a high green coverage rate and hierarchical landscape realms on a medical campus contribute to weakening the institutional atmosphere of the hospital and reducing environmental stress. As one focus group participant commented about Hospital A, "when first entering the campus you won't feel a hospital; it's like a resort." Both hospital buildings were designed in a way that is highly transparent to the exterior, thereby strengthening the people–nature connection and interactions. High visibility and direct accessibility ensured the more frequent use of the garden space. A greenspace closer to the building entrance or a traffic hub with a high volume of internal and external circulations was typically more known by people and more frequently visited. The most successful garden from both hospitals—namely, the Dining Patio (B-1) at Hospital B—is located in the front of the main medical building, with direct connections to two main entrances (the hospital main entrance and entrance to the Women and Children's Hospital) and a staff entrance. This garden is strategically connected with the campus trail system and the visitor and staff parking lot. In addition, the garden is internally adjacent to the cafeteria and coffee shop and close to the hospital gift shop, which makes this garden highly visible and accessible by visitors. Because of its successful location, this garden is a lively place that constantly attracts a wide range of users throughout the day.

Although the Children's ED Therapeutic Garden (B-2) at Hospital B is also located near a building entrance, it is rarely used by patients. Staff members occasionally use the garden for lunch or an informal meeting. The focus group participants confirmed that the space is inadequately used because of a lack of direct physical access from the interiors of the main medical buildings. The nearby wellness center building is currently occupied by another health system that provides outpatient and specialty care, meaning Garden B-2 is located on the edge of the main campus of Hospital B. In addition, visitors to the Children's ED are usually young patients with critical conditions, and patients and family members are usually not able to stay outside long.

The Main Courtyard (A-3) at Hospital A is close to the MOB entrance and the hospital gift shop, but is only used occasionally by a small group of staff members during their lunch or coffee breaks. It is a small courtyard and can easily get crowded. One participant in the focus group described it as a "fishbowl" feeling when she sat in the garden, as if she were being stared at by people inside. A sign on the door to the garden (i.e., "No Exit") is intended to remind visitors that there is no other exit in the courtyard, yet it has caused confusion for some visitors as they are not sure they are allowed to use the space. One focus group participant who works at the gift shop near the courtyard noted that she fielded frequent inquiries from visitors and members about the purpose of the garden and "who is it for."

Both hospitals have rooftop gardens/terraces, and they all serve as light wells and natural view providers, but are not extensively used physically. For Hospital A, the rooftop garden is dedicated to the women's and children's units; it is a secured zone, meaning the public is not able to enter. The garden does not allow any physical access, except for authorized people to maintain the landscape. These factors have contributed to much lower visibility and accessibility for this rooftop garden at Hospital A, and it is visible from only a limited number of patient rooms and the upper-level rehabilitation rooms. During Hospital A's focus group discussions, many participants were not aware of the existence of this rooftop garden. Meanwhile, at Hospital B, a series of rooftop gardens provide abundant natural light to the infant and pediatric wards. As the NICU nursing manager explained during the focus group, natural light is very important to help develop premature infants' rhythm in NICU, and it is also helpful for other patients to regulate their circadian cycle. To improve the usage of Hospital B's rooftop gardens, some focus group participants—mainly nurses—suggested adding attractive design elements, such as colorful species, decorative wall elements, or a water feature, to make the space a destination. However, other participants, represented by the maintenance staff, expressed concerns about maintaining a water feature and complex plantings in a rooftop environment. All relevant groups—from the administrator and designer to the end users and maintenance team—must communicate and make great efforts to ensure that a rooftop garden functions well and is actively used.

Notes

1. Reuben Rainey commented on the healing effects of nature and modernist architecture in an email communication with the book author in 2021.
2. This study was funded by the Landscape Architecture Foundation 2017 Case Study Investigation Program (LAF-CSI 2017). Details can be found in two publications in the Landscape Performance Series (Jiang & Kaljevic, 2017a, 2017b) and the article published in the *Journal of Therapeutic Horticulture* (Jiang, Staloch, & Kaljevic, 2018).

References

20th Century Architecture. (n.d.). Paimio Sanatorium. http://architecture-history. org/architects/architects/aalto/objects/1928%E2%80%931929,%20Paimio%20 Sanatorium,%20Tuberculosis%20sanatorium%20and%20staff%20housing,%20 Paimio,%20Finland.html

Aalto, A. (1932). Sanatorium i Paimio, Finland [Paimio Sanatorium, Finland]. *Byggmästaren [The Master Builder], 14*(5), 80–83.

Aalto, A. (1997). The humanizing of architecture. In G. Schildt (Ed.), *Alvar Aalto in his own words* (pp. 102–107). Otava. (Original work published in The Technology Review 1940.)

Arnold, D. (2013). *The spaces of the hospital: Spatiality and urban change in London 1680–1820*. Routledge.

Campbell, M. (2005). What tuberculosis did for modernism: The influence of a curative environment on modernist design and architecture. *Medical History, 49*(4), 463–488.

Cooper Marcus, C. (2007). Healing gardens in hospitals. *Interdisciplinary Design and Research e-Journal, 1*(1), 1–27.

Cooper Marcus, C., & Francis, C. (Eds). (1998). *People places: Design guidelines for urban open space* (2nd ed.). John Wiley & Sons, Inc.

Cooper Marcus, C., & Sachs, N. A. (2013). Gardens in the healthcare facilities: Steps toward evaluation and certification. *World Health Design, 6*(6), 76–83.

Cooper Marcus, C., & Sachs, N. A. (2014). *Therapeutic landscapes: An evidence-based approach to designing healing gardens and restorative outdoor spaces*. John Wiley & Sons.

Davis, B. E. (2011). Rooftop hospital gardens for physical therapy: A post-occupancy evaluation. *Health Environments Research & Design Journal, 4*(3), 14–43.

Facility Guidelines Institute. (2014). *Guidelines for design and construction of hospitals and outpatient facilities*. American Hospital Association.

Gallos, P. L. (1985). *Cure cottages of Saranac Lake: Architecture and history of a pioneer health resort*. Historic Saranac Lake.

Gerlach-Spriggs, N., Kaufman, R. E., & Warner, S. B. (1998). *Restorative gardens: The healing landscape*. Yale University Press.

Gerteis, M., Edgman-Levitan, S., Daley, J., & Delbanco, T. L. (1993). *Through the patient's eyes: Understanding and promoting patient-centered care.*. John Wiley & Sons, Inc.

Grahn, A. (2015, August 6). *Tuberculosis sanitariums: Reminders of the white plague*. National Trust for Historic Preservation. https://savingplaces.org/stories/tuberculosis-sanitariums-reminders-of-the-white-plaque#.YC7E1BNKiu4

Heath, Y., & Gifford, R. (2001). Post-occupancy evaluation of therapeutic gardens in a multi-level care facility for the aged. *Activities, Adaptation & Aging, 25*(2), 21–43.

Heikinheimo, M. (2016). *Architecture and technology: Alvar Aalto's Paimio Sanatorium*. Aalto University.

Heikinheimo, M. (2018a). *Paimio Sanatorium*. http://www.paimiosanatorium.fi/

Heikinheimo, M. (2018b). Paimio Sanatorium under construction. *Arts, 7*(4), 78. http://dx.doi.org/10.3390/arts7040078

Heikkonen, N. (2016). *Paimio Sanatorium Conservation Management Plan 2016*. Alvar Aalto Foundation.

Hickman, C. (2013). *Therapeutic landscapes: A history of English hospital gardens since 1800*. Manchester University Press.

Historic England. (2017, December). *Health and welfare buildings: Listing selection guide*. https://historicengland.org.uk/images-books/publications/dlsg-health-welfare-buildings/heag112-health-and-welfare-lsg/

Hobday, R. A. (1997). Sunlight therapy and solar architecture. *Medical History, 41*(4), 455–472.

Jiang, S., & Kaljevic, S. (2017a). *Owensboro Health Regional Hospital (Landscape performance series)*. Landscape Architecture Foundation. https://doi.org/10.31353/cs1210

Jiang, S., & Kaljevic, S. (2017b). *Virtua Voorhees Hospital (Landscape performance series)*. Landscape Architecture Foundation. https://doi.org/10.31353/cs1190

Jiang, S., Staloch, K., & Kaljevic, S. (2018). Opportunities and barriers to using hospital gardens: Comparative post occupancy evaluations of healthcare landscape environments. *Journal of Therapeutic Horticulture, 28*(2), 23–56.

Kim, H. (2009). Alvar Aalto and humanizing of architecture. *Journal of Asian Architecture and Building Engineering, 8*(1), 9–16. 10.3130/jaabe.8.9

King, A. (1966). Hospital planning: Revised thoughts on the origin of the pavilion principle in England. *Medical History, 10*(4), 360–373.

Le Corbusier (1985). *Towards a new architecture* (F. Etchells, Trans.). Dover Publications. (Original published 1931.)

Martini, M., Gazzaniga, V., Behzadifar, M., Bragazzi, N. L., & Barberis, I. (2018). The history of tuberculosis: The social role of sanatoria for the treatment of tuberculosis in Italy between the end of the 19th century and the middle of the 20th. *Journal of Preventive Medicine and Hygiene, 59*(4), E323.

Nightingale, F. (1860). *Notes on nursing: What it is, and what it is not*. William Carter. https://en.wikisource.org/wiki/Notes_on_Nursing:_What_It_Is,_and_What_It_Is_Not

Nightingale, F. (1863). *Notes on hospitals*. Longman, Green, Longman, Roberts, and Green. https://archive.org/details/notesonhospital01nighgoog/page/n2/mode/2up

Overy, P. (2007). *Light, air and openness: Modern architecture between the wars.*. Thames and Hudson Ltd.

Pasha, S. (2013). Barriers to garden visitation in children's hospitals. *Health Environments Research & Design Journal, 6*(4), 76–96.

Preiser, W., Rabinowitz, H. Z., & White, E. T. (1988). *Post occupancy evaluation*. Routledge.

Sachs, N. (2017). *The healthcare garden evaluation toolkit: A standardized method for evaluation, research, and design of gardens in healthcare facilities* [Doctoral dissertation, Texas A & M University]. http://hdl.handle.net/1969.1/173045

Sherman, S. A., Varni, J. W., Ulrich, R. S., & Malcarne, V. L. (2005). Post-occupancy evaluation of healing gardens in a pediatric cancer center. *Landscape and Urban Planning, 73*(2–3), 167–183.

Strickland, T. (2017). Passive and active: Public space at the McMaster Health Sciences Centre, 1972. In S. Schrank, & D. Ekici (Eds.), *Healing spaces, modern architecture, and the body* (pp. 203–223). Routledge.

Theodore, D. (2017). The decline of the hospital as a healing machine. In S. Schrank, & D. Ekici (Eds.), *Healing spaces, modern architecture, and the body* (pp. 186–202). Routledge.

Thompson, J. D., & Goldin, G. (1975). *The hospital: A social and architectural history*. Yale University Press.

Tomes, N. (1994). *The art of asylum-keeping: Thomas Story Kirkbride and the origins of American psychiatry*. University of Pennsylvania Press.

Ulrich, R. P., Quan, X., Zimring, C. P., Joseph, A., & Choudhary, R. (September, 2004). *The role of the physical environment in the hospital of the 21st century: A once-in-a-lifetime opportunity*. The Center for Health Design. https://www.healthdesign.org/knowledge-repository/role-physical-environment-hospital-21st-century-once-lifetime-opportunity

Verderber, S. (2003). Architecture for health-2050: An international perspective. *The Journal of Architecture, 8*(3), 281–302.

Verderber, S., & Fine, D. J. (2000). *Healthcare architecture in an era of radical transformation.* Yale University Press.

Warren, P. (2006). The evolution of the sanatorium: The first half-century, 1854–1904. *Canadian Bulletin of Medical History, 23*(2), 457–476.

Whitehouse, S., Varni, J. W., Seid, M., Cooper Marcus, C., Ensberg, M. J., Jacobs, J. R., & Mehlenbeck, R. S. (2001). Evaluating a children's hospital garden environment: Utilization and consumer satisfaction. *Journal of Environmental Psychology, 21*(3), 301–314.

5 Transparency and Transparent Spaces in Hospital Design: From Theories to Practices

The mainstream trend of humanistic care in the 21st century advocates for humanized hospital design. Greenspaces and the consequential health benefits in contemporary hospitals have been discussed in previous chapters, together with some persistent issues identified regarding the usage situations of different types of greenspaces. Low visibility and accessibility as well as the disconnected indoor–outdoor relationship hinder the effective people–nature engagement in hospital environments. Therefore, it is necessary to reinvent the relationship among the site, landscape, and building and blur the "often stark, abrupt line of demarcation" between the interior and exterior environments (Verderber, 2010).

The term *theraserialization* is a hybrid assemblage of the words therapeutic and serialize coined by Stephen Verderber (2010). It refers to a continuum of indoor to outdoor space consciously designed in support of biophilic environmental design principles. As asserted by Loftness and Snyder (2008, p. 119), "Biophilic design recognizes that the line between indoors and outdoors must be rethought; that indoor rooms must communicate with outdoor rooms; that windows must become doors." *Theraserialization* entails the interpretation of space as being serialized, layered, collaged, superimposed, transparent, and fluid. It is about the creation of serialized space from the public to semipublic, semiprivate, and private. It is also about the spaces in between and about illusion. Verderber (2010) identified five strategies to break down the needless barriers between a hospital and the natural environment, including water, roofscaping, surrogates, healing gardens, and transparency, in a two-way continuum between the interior and exterior. "By peeling away, or dematerializing, the physical and symbolic barriers that cut the interior of a building off from the outside world, its true 'nature' can be revealed and the building can breathe" (p. 52).

Transparency supports *theraserialization* and the inside-out spatial communication. However, an optically translucent condition alone is not necessarily equivalent to a hospital's *theraserialized* configuration. Full height windows that connect a clinic's waiting room with the outdoors cannot succeed in this regard if waiting room occupants must look out directly onto

DOI: 10.4324/9781003122180-5

the monotonous pavement or a parking lot. In contrast, if the windows in this same room overlook a pleasant garden or natural context, the visual effect can be perceived as restorative, soothing, and therefore far more preferable (Jiang & Verderber, 2016).

Transparency as a school of thought in modernist architecture was first initiated by Collin Rowe and Robert Slutzky (1963) and frequently discussed in the context of residential buildings. Hospitals are extreme complex buildings, and their functional complicity is comparable to a small city (Allison, 2007). This chapter deciphers the logic and feasibility of applying transparency in large institutional buildings, such as hospitals, through an urban design approach. A preliminary pattern language of transparent spaces, through windows and materials as well as spatial organization, is suggested in hospital design. A combination of literal and phenomenal transparency offers possibilities to achieve *theraserialization* and an optimized person–nature engagement in large hospitals.

Phenomenal Transparency and Spatial Continuity as an Urban Approach[1]

Transparency: From Rowe and Slutzky to Hoesli

Colin Rowe and Robert Slutzky's (1963) "Transparency: Literal and Phenomenal" was a ground-breaking seminal text influencing architecture and art in the second half of the 20th century. For Rowe and Slutzky, transparency implies more than the inherent optical characteristic of material—namely, glass; it refers to a simultaneous perception of elements in different spatial locations. Inspired by György Kepes' attempt to overcome the disintegration of vision from space, which can be traced back to the fragmentation of knowledge in the late 18th century, Rowe and Slutzky (1963) sought to understand its phenomenal interpretation. Kepes (1944) elucidated the ambiguity between vision and space with reference to an alternative perceptual quality that he called "transparency." In Kepes' view:

> If one sees two or more figures partly overlapping one another, and each of them claims for itself the common overlapped part, then one is confronted with a contradiction of spatial dimensions. To resolve this contradiction, one must assume the presence of a new optical quality. The figures are endowed with transparency; that is, they are able to interpenetrate without an optical destruction of each other. [Transparency,] however, implies more than an optical characteristic; it implies a broader spatial order. Transparency means a simultaneous perception of different spatial locations. Space not only recedes but also fluctuates in a continuous activity. The position of the transparent figures has equivocal meaning as one sees each figure now as the closer, now as the further one. (Kepes, 1944, p. 77)

Phenomenal transparency describes the perceptual quality that allows the human mind to discern the underlying spatial organization of a built environment (Oechslin, 1997). To distinguish their phenomenal interpretation from the literal transparency (i.e., being pervious to light and air), Rowe and Slutzky (1963) associated the perceptual quality of architecture with visual arts and Cubist paintings. Interpreting the painting *La Sarraz* by László Moholy-Nagy, a visual artist and professor in the Bauhaus school, Rowe and Slutzky pointed out that spatial depth was achieved through a pure color pigmentation and the superimposition of geometrical elements in different dimensions. Despite the fact that the composition is completely devoid of any component reminiscent of nature and the paint is physically transparent, for Rowe and Slutzky, this picture still recalled the traditional pre-Cubist technique of "foreground, middleground and background" (p. 48) and allowed for only one way of reading (Figure 5.1 left). In their view, all Moholy-Nagy achieved was to look at outer space through a private, secluded window. On the other hand, Fernand Léger's *Three Faces* presented a shallow, abstracted space "charged with an equivocal depth" (p. 48) open to alternative readings (Figure 5.1 right). Léger's picture is fundamentally composed of three segments in opaque colors. In this composition, the painter successfully imagined some orthogonal contours to align the organic forms, abstracted artifacts, and geometrical shapes in these three segments. Briefly, whereas Léger pondered the spatial relations among the pictorial objects in his composition, Moholy-Nagy largely dealt with material and light (Jiang & Ersoy, 2017; Rowe & Slutzky, 1997) (Figure 5.1).

In terms of architecture, Rowe and Slutzky (1963) were similarly critical of the way in which transparency was literally associated with the optical characteristics of a glazed wall. Regarding literal transparency, the building in their mind was the Dessau Bauhaus (1925–1926) designed by Walter Gropius. Similar to Moholy-Nagy, Gropius was preoccupied with the chromatic and optical aberrations that the material and light generated more than

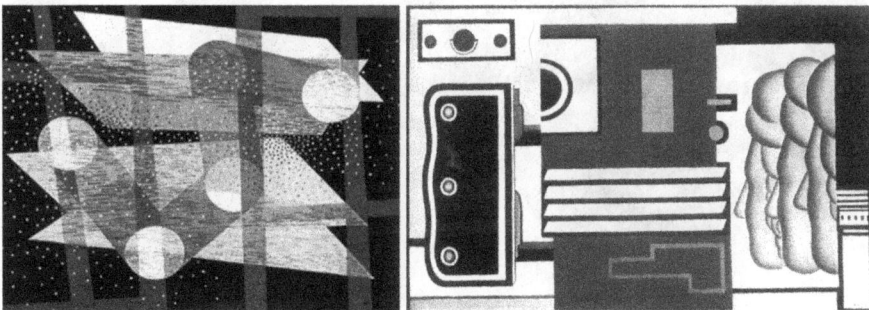

Figure 5.1 Comparison between *La Sarraz* by László Moholy-Nagy (left) and *Three Faces* by Fernand Léger (right)

the spatial continuity. In their view, the alternative comparable with Léger's *Three Faces* was Villa Stein in Garches (1927) by Le Corbusier and Pierre Jeanneret. The villa's irregular façade and broken grid presented to Rowe and Slutzky an analogous spatial stratification. The significant subtraction on the second-floor plan of the villa gives a depth to its flat façade and divides the building into volumes. However, unorthodox internal divisions and external projections that act like contours deny this division by setting up dialogue among architectural elements in both vertical and horizontal directions. For Rowe and Slutzky, what endowed this building with the quality of phenomenal transparency was its perceptual ambiguity, which stimulates one to hunt for an underlying spatial order (Rowe & Slutzky, 1997, pp. 30–32).

Bernhard Hoesli, a professor of architecture at ETH Zurich, embraced Rowe and Slutzky's approach and sought to extend phenomenal transparency to a design method and analytical tool. Hoesli drew on the technique of axonometric drawing to illustrate and clarify the "shallow space" in Le Corbusier's cubist eyes. In his view, Le Corbusier's *Nature morte a la pile d'assiettes* (1920) and Villa Stein (1926–1928) shared the same formal organization and could be read as being composed of a series of layers in the shape of elevation sections. Seemingly, Le Corbusier connected the vertical spaces "through a common expanse of air [which] has the effect not only of optically increasing the size of small rooms but also of generating ambiguous spatial relations" (Hoesli, 1997a, p. 72). Villa Stein represents a transparent system of spatial relations (Figure 5.2).

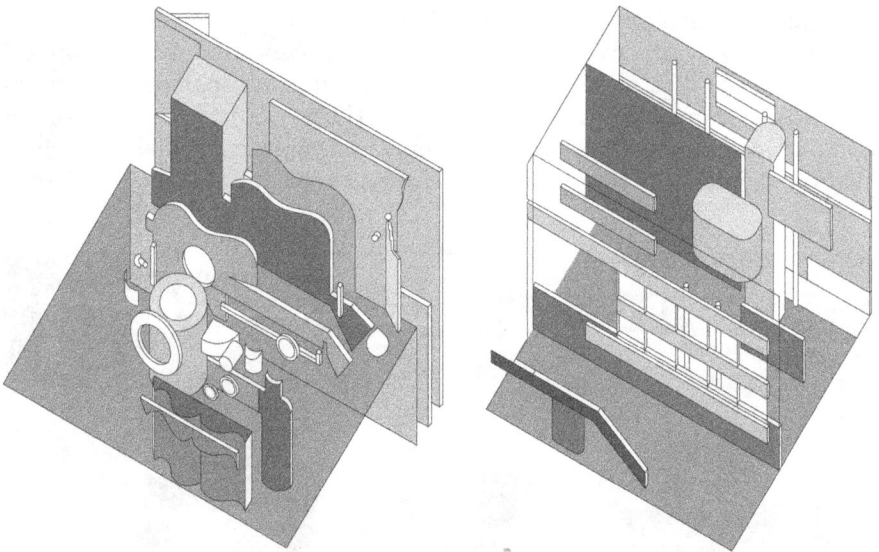

Figure 5.2 Comparative axonometric analyses of the spatial layering in Le Corbusier's painting *Nature morte a la pile d'assiettes* and the Villa Stein at Garches (Hoesli, 1997a)

Source: Drawn by Shan Jiang and Udday Datta

Phenomenal Transparency and Spatial Continuity

Phenomenal transparency transcends the use of pure vision to depict a distance and static view that occurs when the body of an observer is at rest. As early as the 19th century, art historian and perceptual psychologist August Schmarsow (1993) brought forth the kinesthetic implications of architecture and advocated that one can project our vision forward into the spatial form by imagining ourselves in motion, by measuring the various dimensions of width and depth, and by attributing to the immobile lines, surfaces, and volumes in the movement of the eyes and muscular sensations. Considering the indissoluble correspondence between architectural space and the eye in motion that Schmarsow stressed, phenomenal transparency can be associated with a spatio-temporal continuity that blurs the boundaries and questions how an enclosure is defined (Jiang & Ersoy, 2017). Le Corbusier's ideas of "free plan" and architectural promenade support this spatio-temporal approach:

> You enter: the architectural spectacle at once offers itself to the eye. You follow an itinerary and the perspectives develop with great variety, developing a play of light on the walls or making pools of shadow. Large windows open up views of the exterior where the architectural unity is reasserted.... (Le Corbusier & Jeanneret, 1937, p. 60)

Adolf Loos, credited as the founder of Rationalism and International Style in modern architecture (Maciuika, 2000), offered an experience of phenomenal transparency and spatial continuity in the interiors of Villa Muller (built in 1930). Loos claimed his architecture was not conceived in plan, but in spaces:

> My architecture is not conceived in plans, but in spaces. I do not design floor plans, facades, sections. I design spaces. For me, there is no ground floor, first floor etc.... For me, there are only contiguous, continual spaces, rooms, anterooms, terraces etc. Stories merge and spaces relate to each other. (Loos, 1930[2])

Leatherbarrow's (2005) analysis of Villa Muller expands on Loos' ideas of spatial continuity:

> Before this room is entered, looking right, the dining room can be seen at the top of a flight of steps, on the left another semi-spiral stairway begins. Straight ahead from the point of arrival on the main level are windows that are open onto the rear garden in the foreground and Prague in the distance. Thus from this point three primary settings are interconnected.... (p. 13)

A Continuum of Indoor–Outdoor Spaces

Wendy Redfield (2005) has pointed out that historians have largely ignored the issue of site in their accounts of many purist villas. The comprehension of Le Corbusier's villas cannot complete without experiencing the continuum of indoor–outdoor spaces. As noted in Flora Samuel's (2010) text, the architectural promenade—the observer's pathway through the built space—as an essential element of Le Corbusier's environmental designs creates a spatial continuity expandable to a vast nature context:

> …a quasi-exterior route through the building, its progress interrupted by the most minimal of glass doors at ground level. These cause a blurring of interior and exterior space, pulling the exterior route into the house and up to the rooftop garden. (p. 11)

Such spatial continuity served modern architects to realign their buildings with nature and to re-sensitize dwellers to their surroundings (Samuel, 2010). Madame Savoye, the client of Villa Savoye, believed in the therapeutic benefits of nature and outdoor leisure and the villa fully integrated interior spaces and nature to let the household experience outdoor leisure efficiently (Figure 5.3). Looking through the floor-to-ceiling window in the living room on the second floor, one can perceive both the domesticated nature on the deck and the wild nature behind the horizontal windows on the exterior wall. The roof garden became a phenomenally transparent space that simultaneously belonged to the villa and performed as an extension of nature (Jiang & Ersoy, 2017).

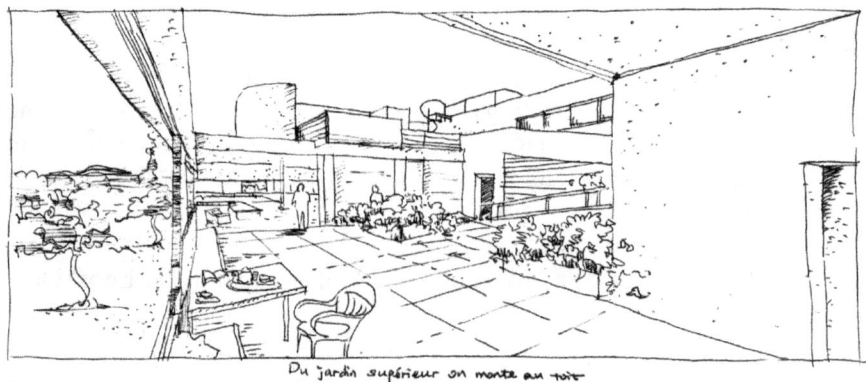

Du jardin supérieur on monte au toit

Figure 5.3 Sketch of Villa Savoye roof garden by Le Corbusier (built between 1928 and 1931), first published in the essay *Savoye Space* by Daniel Naegele (2001), *Harvard Design Magazine*, No. 15, Fall 2001

Source: Adapted from Le Corbusier (1929), first published in the essay *Savoye Space* by Daniel Naegele (2001), *Harvard Design Magazine*, No. 15, Fall 2001. Redrawn by Shan Jiang.

Frank Lloyd Wright was another advocate of the continuum between the natural and built environment. Wright's Prairie Style usually favored an open ground plan contained within a horizontal format comprising low profiles of roofs and bounding walls that were deliberately integrated into the natural external (Frampton, 2007). Wright described this as "breaking the box" (1955, p. 77). Inspired by Wright's architecture, Van Doesburg explained that "new architecture had opened the walls of the building and thereby eliminated any separation between inside and outside, the room and the garden, allowing the one to pass over into the other and a new openness to emerge" (Leatherbarrow, 2004, p. 97). Taking advantage of the climate conditions of Southern California, Richard Neutra and Rudolph Schindler—two of Wright's apprentices—designed buildings transparent to nature that appeared to grow out of their natural settings (Sternberg, 2009).

Neutra was very sensitive to the natural world and he believes in a "bio-realism" design philosophy, which emphasizes the relationship between the physiological and psychological realities of human existence (Hille, 2011). His writings and designs revealed how he saw human life enmeshed in a network of relationships between the built and natural environment (Leatherbarrow, 2004). He wrote:

Man is always in the middle of something—this ineluctable presence, enveloping and permeating our lives, is called the environment. It ties us together. It determines who we are, how we feel and what our outlook is. Of primordial vintage...the environment, depending on how sensitively we manage its complement of resources, can either erode or strengthen our sanity and civility, and these are as essential to survival, in any meaningful and lasting human sense, as clean air and water. (Neutra & Marlin, 1989, p. 5)

Neutra was explicit about the health benefits of well-planned architecture and the importance of nature in health. He usually interweaved literal and phenomenal transparency into his design work aimed to optimize daylight, ventilation, and people's contacts with nature from the public health perspectives. The most representative example of Neutra's desire to overcome the separation between architecture and its natural surroundings was his transformation of external walls into movable partitions, allowing the interior space to flow out into the exterior (Leatherbarrow, 2004). One can easily perceive nature through the phenomenally transparent components—namely, the partitions, the frames, and the seamless glass. Additional design language in Neutra's work includes the post-and-beam construction for openness and flexibility, cantilevered planar walls for spatial interpenetration, expansive areas of glass for visual transparency, and patios and gardens for outdoor activities close to nature (Hille, 2011). As evident in the design of Singleton House (opened in 1959), water flowed indoors, and the interior was canopied by the trees; one's line of sight can easily penetrate

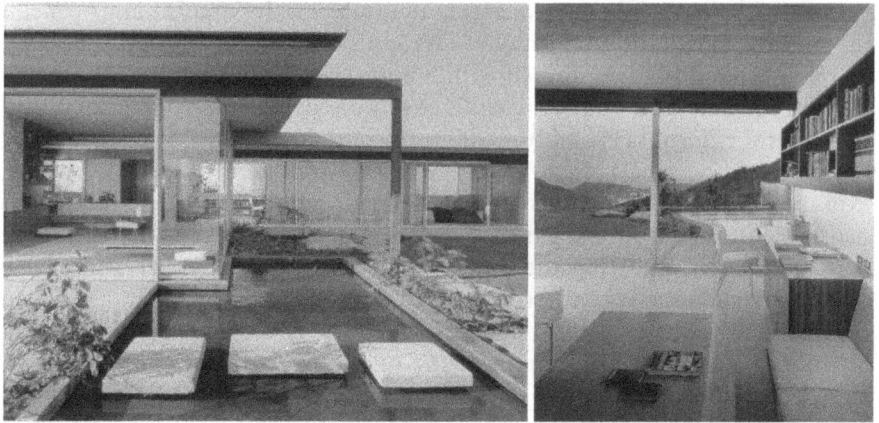

Figure 5.4 Singleton House exterior (left) and interior (right), designed by Richard
Neutra in 1959

Source: Photographer for both images: Julius Shulman © J. Paul Getty Trust. Getty Research
Institute, Los Angeles (2004.R.10; Job 2926)

the entire place and ultimately end in nature, thereby creating the illusion
that the indoors was a part of the outside and the outside was an extension
of the interior (Figure 5.4).

Although best known for his unique designs of modern houses in southern California, Neutra has designed a number of institutional buildings,
particularly schools, under the influence of the Open-Air School for Healthy
Child movement that emerged in the early 1920s in Europe (Hille, 2011).
Jan Duiker, the original designer of Zonnestraal Sanatorium (Figure 4.2),
was also the forerunner to design open-air schools, a viable alternative to
the sanatorium where children could receive both treatment and education.
The Open-Air Schools' notable qualities include the substantial sense of
openness and interconnectivity, especially in the relationship of the classrooms to the out-of-doors, the transparency, and extreme delicacy of the
window-wall enclosure system (Hille, 2011). In many of Neutra and partners' school design projects, window walls, sheltered patios, and numerous
semi-public transitions extended the classroom activities into the surrounding landscape. In the Corona Avenue School (designed in 1935) project,
each classroom features a large sliding window wall that opens directly
to the outside, transforming the interior space into a porch and a courtyard that functioned as an "open-air" classroom. In the UCLA Nursery-
Kindergarten and Elementary School (designed in 1957) project, Neutra
and Robert Alexander created window walls, sheltered patios, and numerous semi-public transitions that extended the classroom activities into the
surrounding landscape. To integrate with the natural surroundings and
encourage indoor–outdoor continuity, courtyards were fully developed as

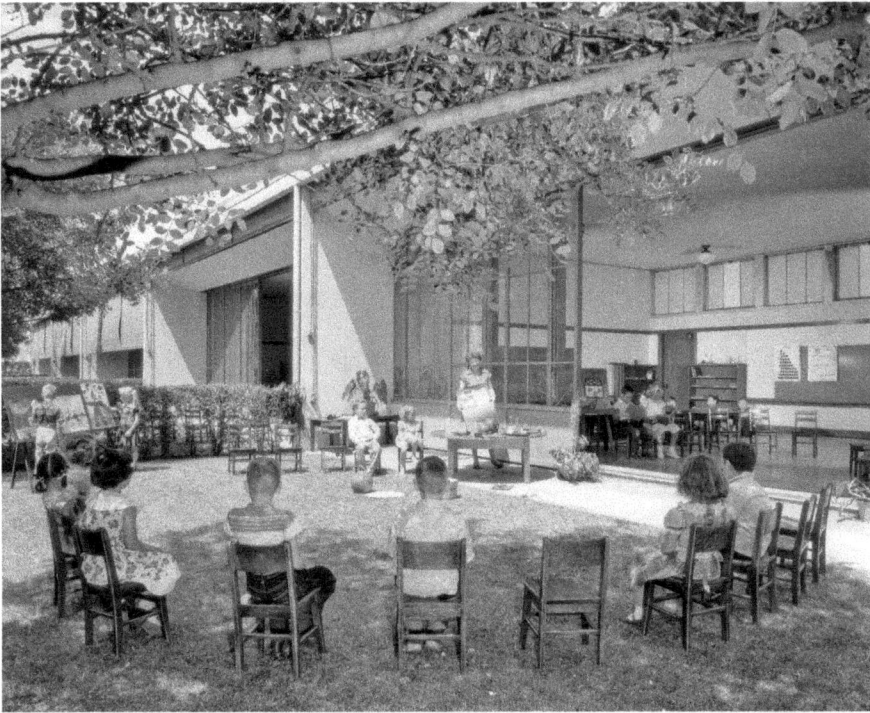

Figure 5.5 Corona Avenue School, Los Angeles, California, designed by Richard
Neutra in 1953

Source: Photographer: Julius Shulman © J. Paul Getty Trust. Getty Research Institute, Los
Angeles (2004.R.10; Job 1545)

outdoor rooms, and mature trees on site were directly incorporated into the
structure's system (Hille, 2011) (Figure 5.5).

Phenomenal Transparency: An Urban Design Approach

Many of the modernist solutions for creating indoor–outdoor spatial continuity became less effective when dealing with large, institutional complexes
rather than intimate spaces such as villas. Phenomenal transparency, a characteristic particular to not only buildings, was further considered applicable
for analyzing the spatial relationship existing in large-scale and even urban
components. Similar spatial continuities exist in urban contexts. As early
as the last decades of the 19th century, Camillo Sitte (1986), an Austrian
architect and urban theorist, elucidated the spatial continuums in the city
context in his book *City Planning according to Artistic Principles*. Sitte was
mainly concerned with the increasingly technical way the contemporary
cities were being designed at the expense of traditional artistic methods.

He traveled throughout European Renaissance and Baroque cities to under-stand how the cities developed and to decode the set of principles used to arrange piazzas. Among the 255 piazzas he observed, Sitte (1986) found that the key element of a successful urban design was the public building surrounded by public squares (Figure 5.6). Churches, then the central components of the parishes, were mostly attached to another building in the same piazza, serving as hinges connecting two or three squares and serving various civic

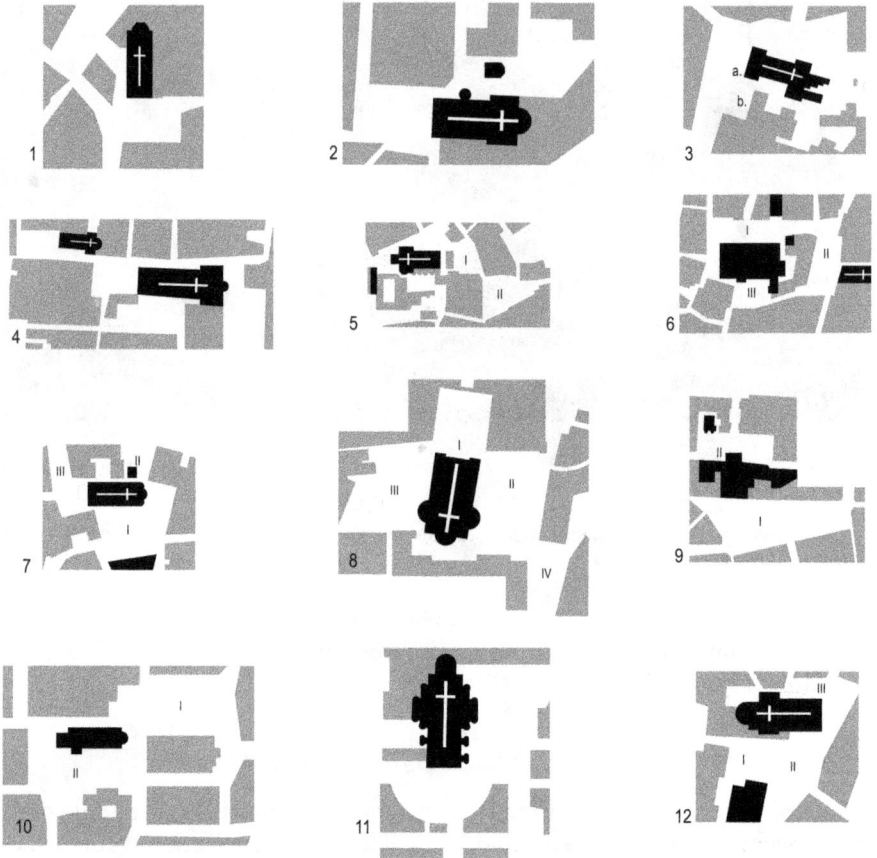

1. PADOUE. Piazza Petrarca | 2. RAVENNE. Piazza del Duomo | 3. NUREMBERG. Place Saint-Eloi. (a) Eglise Saint-Eloi. (b) Gymnase. 4. LUCQUES. Piazza Grande | 5. GIMIGNANO. (I) Piazza del Duomo. (II) Piazza della Cisterna. | 6. VICENCE. (I) Piazza del Signori. (II) Pescheria. (III) Piazza della Biava. | 7. MODENE. (I). Piazza Grande. (II). Piazza Torre. (III). Piazza della Legna. | 8. SALZBOURG. (I). Place du Dome. (II). Place de la Residence. (III). Place du Chapitre. (IV). Place Mozart. | 9. COLOGNE. (I) Vieux Marche. (II). Place de l'Hotel de Ville. | 10. BRUNSWICK. (I) Place de Marche. (II). Place Saint-Martin. | 11. CATANE. S. Nicolo. | 12. PEROUSE. (I) Piazza del Vescovado. (II) Piazza di S Lorenzo. (III) Piazza del Papa.

Figure 5.6 Successful forms of urban public open spaces discussed in Sitte's (1986) original study

Source: Drawn by Shan Jiang and Udday Datta

purposes (Sitte, 1986, p. 19). Churches belonged to several squares simultaneously while serving as an intersection and phenomenally transparent component among them (Jiang & Ersoy, 2017).

According to Hoesli's (1997b) interpretation, exterior open spaces and interiors can be connected and somehow transformed by phenomenal transparency. As illustrated by Hoesli, depending on the degree of enclosure that the space boundary exerts, the inside space can be felt as part of the outside; hence, space becomes continuous and fluid. Urban fabric is a spontaneously developed organic system that allowed for intersections among buildings and open spaces. In this system, there is no explicit front figure and background relationship, such as with a palace in the middle of an extensive landscape. The continuous flow of people from one built environment to another inevitably involves phenomenal transparency between the spaces. Porticos were once the common transition spaces between interior–exterior areas, and streets could be an extension of shops and homes; they were tightly attached to the buildings surrounding a square and partially open to the piazza at the same time. As a result, people sitting in a café in a portico could easily become confused about whether they are indoors or outdoors. Thus, architecture demonstrated the capacity to make piazzas and streets outdoor rooms (Rudofsky, 1969).

Architects throughout history have recognized the analogy between buildings and cities. Leon Battista Alberti was the first one to make this analogy: "Compartition is the process of dividing up the site into yet smaller units, so that the building may be considered as being made up of close- fitting smaller buildings…" (Alberti, 1988, p. 8). In this sense, "if the city is like some large house, and the house is in turn like some small city, cannot the various parts of the house… be considered miniature buildings?" (Alberti, 1988, p. 23). Alison Smithson (1991), an English architect and member of Team Ten, argued that this analogy was no longer coherent in modern life conditions. However, certain types of institutional buildings with a massive scale, like general hospitals and medical centers, could still be described as a small city due to the complexity in their programs. David Allison, a scholar and distinguished educator in healthcare architecture, suggested that a hospital can be analogous to a small city as it contains types of places that accommodate activities and experiences similar to those in urban life—namely, birth, death, healthcare, work, exchange, learning, research, and worship (Allison, 2007).

Lessons Learned from the Venice Hospital

As urban approaches became inevitable in the planning and design of such architecture, phenomenal transparency and interior–exterior spatial continuity could be adopted for successful designs. The Venice Hospital (deigned between 1964 and 1965), an avant-garde modern hospital designed by Le Corbusier and Guillermo Jullian de la Fuente, sustained the intentions

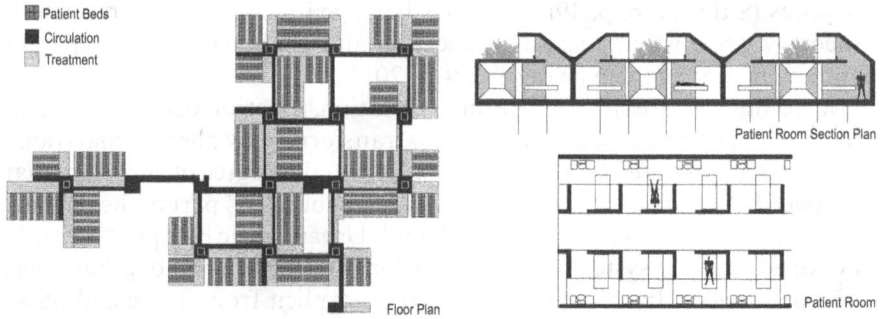

Figure 5.7 The patient room, patient unit, and spatial configuration in the original plan of the Venice Hospital by Le Corbusier and Guillermo Jullian de la Fuente, designed in 1965

Source: Drawn by Shan Jiang and Udday Datta

of seamlessly imbedding a giant structure into the existing urban fabric. Although it was an unrealized project, and despite the failure of the patient room design (monotonous patient rooms with low ceilings and no windows on the sidewalls, with only a skylight included to introduce daylight), the layout of the hospital illustrated how public open spaces and the architectural interiors interweaved with each other. The program was a 1,200-bed medical center initially designed on the site of a former slaughterhouse in the San Giobbe neighborhood in Cannaregio. The first phase of the design took place in 1965 and, after Le Corbusier's death, Guillermo Jullian de la Fuente took primary responsibility for the design. Patient rooms were located on the upper story; 28 patient rooms and 3 corridors comprised a square unit (Figure 5.7). The ground floor, housing other medical services, was built on pilotis and accessible by boats (Jiang & Ersoy, 2017).

The Venice Hospital was frequently interpreted as a Mat building (Sarkis et al., 2001) and compared to Candilis, Josic, and Woods' design of the Free University of Berlin (Frampton, 2007). However, Jullian de la Fuente strongly resisted the categorization of the Venice Hospital into Mat building typology. Mahnaz Shah's analysis sustained Jullian de la Fuente's argument that the Venice Hospital design was based on its site-specific context and was far more complicated than Mat building typology, which was "a more generic solution to mega structures in architectural discourses" (Shah, 2013, p. 168).

The urban morphology of Venice influenced the configuration of the Venice Hospital. The hospital was designed to extend the urban fabric of the historic city while simultaneously turning it into flexible quasi-urban interior environments (Psarra, 2012). As Pablo Allard speculated,

the plan reads as a regular series of quadrangular areas, each structured around a small 'square' and connected by axial 'street' corridors to the other units in the same level and to other floors by elongated ramps that ran parallel to the 'street.' (Sarkis et al., 2001, p. 26)

Two elements contributed to the spatial continuity between buildings and the external nature: pilotis and patios. "The space of the pilotis forms a shaded region in which the reflections of sunlight on water would create continuous movement..." (Addington et al., 2001, p. 69). Meanwhile, patios were more than just the static result of a solid carved out to gain light and air; they also formed a series of phenomenally transparent spaces in urban Venice in both a physical and spiritual way. The "free plan" principle allowed the interweaving of open, semi-open, and closed spaces to set up a continuity among the historic urban fabric, water, and open air. As Allard (2001) commented:

> Following the explorations started at the 1964 Carpenter Center in Cambridge, the interactions of inside and outside space are consciously activated by means of layers of transparencies and visual fluidity that dissolve the contextual difficulties faced in Harvard building by dematerializing the facades and the limits of the envelope, and projecting the envelope, and projecting the surrounding buildings as the ultimate façade. In Venice, this effect is intensified by the shimmering reflections of the sun on the water and its projections on the slabs, walls, glassed surfaces, and pilotis. (p. 31)

More recently, the interpretation of the spatial continuity and hospital–city encounter in the Venice Hospital has been empirically tested. Space syntax as a spatial analytical tool was able to evaluate the configuration and network of relationships, both spatially and socially, in architecture or urban planning (Setola & Borgianni, 2016). Psarra (2012) conducted a space syntax analysis on the Venice Hospital plans and found that the entire building is well integrated in terms of both its internal organization and its relationship with the exterior. As analyzed by Psarra (2012), the high level of spatial continuity was achieved through the extensive horizontal and vertical links in the design, which established large-scale spatial connects on each floor and from the top to the ground level. In order to let daylight reach the inner parts of the Venice Hospital, the spatial configuration included a series of courtyards and patios traversed by pathways and bridges. The axial visibility analysis revealed that the square-shaped center of each patient room unit in the Venice Hospital served as the joining point where the structure of visibility intersects with the structure of movement. The unit centers were adjacent to the decentered nursing stations with dematerialized boundaries, meaning they were not bound by boundaries on all four sides, but instead open to voids and gardens on at least two sides. Such a configuration is well analogizable to the interconnected streets and squares of the city of Venice (Psarra, 2012).

A Preliminary Pattern Language of Transparent Spaces in Hospitals[3]

Integrating transparent spaces, both literally and phenomenally, has been considered an effective strategy in promoting people–nature contact in hospitals. Inspired by the architectural typology studies by Christopher Alexander and his colleagues (1977), a preliminary pattern language of transparent spaces is suggested in this section. The term *pattern* refers to components, items, and design characteristics interchangeable that have happened and can be repeatedly reapplied in the built environment. According to Alexander and colleagues' (1977) original description, "each pattern describes a problem which occurs over and over again in our environment, and then describes the core of the solution to that problem, in such a way that you can use this solution a million times over..." (p. X). Inspired by *The Timeless Way of Building* (Alexander, 1979) and *A Pattern Language* (Alexander et al., 1977), Martha Tyson (1998) translated behavioral research to design patterns that are applicable to therapeutic outdoor environments, particularly those for the elderly and disabled. Tyson (1998, p. 43) described patterns as "the elements of the language of design. Patterns are like the individual words or phrases that are combined when creating prose or poetry." Also inspired by Alexander, in the book *With People in Mind*, Rachel Kaplan and co-authors (1998) adopted a pattern language format in the design and management of everyday nature. The patterns suggested the relationship between the aspects of the environment and how people experience or react to them. Kaplan et al. (1998) provided possible solutions to some recurring situations in environmental design.

Next this chapter discusses each newly developed pattern, including its title and a brief introduction, illustration, inspiration, and possible design applications in the hospital context. Several texts serve as the source of inspirations. *A Pattern Language* (Alexander et al., 1977) served as the major source of inspiration, particularly the global patterns in towns and buildings that give shape to groups of buildings and the lands in between. Other sources include the types and locations of therapeutic landscapes in healthcare from *Therapeutic Landscapes* by Cooper Marcus and Sachs (2014) and the discussion about *theraserialization* by Verderber (2010).

Pattern 1: Hierarchy of Landscape Realms

This pattern describes the hierarchic green open spaces on a medical campus. Landscape and nature content can be most effective when experienced as a hierarchy of greenspaces traversing private, semi-public, and public spaces. The three primary user constituencies of a hospital—namely, patients, visitors/families, and staff—can benefit from this strategy.

Patterns from Alexander et al. (1977):

- 30—Activity nodes
- 31—Promenade

- 98—Circulation realms
- 108—Connected buildings
- 114—Hierarchy of open space
- 131—The Flow through rooms

Pattern 2: Courtyards that Breathe

This pattern describes the type of low-rise, large building blocks with multiple holes of courtyards. Cooper Marcus and Sachs (2014) described a variety of courtyards that are subtly different. Irregular shapes of building footprints could enclose courtyards with different degrees of openness. Building units grouped in a rough circle around an outdoor space can generate the type of "hole-in-a-donut" garden, as a central gathering hub that converges and directs routes connecting the surrounding building units (Cooper Marcus & Sachs, 2014).
   Patterns from Alexander et al. (1977):

- 60—Accessible green
- 61—Small public squares
- 115—Courtyards which live
- 128—Indoor sunlight
- 129—Common areas at the heart
- 171—Tree places
- 177—Vegetable garden

Pattern 3: Vertical Gardens and Cutouts

In the previous pattern, the focus was to carve out volumes to open up the building envelope. Here, the emphasis is on vertical cutouts, slices, and perforations on building exteriors and sections. In the case of mid- and high-rise healthcare facilities with narrow footprints on dense sites, this process can yield a variety of openings and indentations in composition, yielding more interesting views, and elevated interior-to-exterior connectivity. Oblique and unusual vistas and views can be maximized in this pattern. A vertical garden on the side of a cutout of this type can be analogized to a piece of Swiss cheese.
   Patterns from Alexander et al. (1977):

- 60—Accessible green
- 95—Building complex
- 96—Number of stories
- 128—Indoor sunlight

Pattern 4: Positive Outdoor Spaces

As Alexander et al. (1977) stated, outdoor spaces merely "left over" between buildings will, in general, not be used. The same could be said of healthcare facilities. In contrast, a hospital that provides a series of inviting,

semi-enclosed outdoor rooms for their users can add to one's sense of protection, safety, and the ability to directly experience the outdoors while
simultaneously feeling connected to adjoining interior spaces. Gardens that
surround and lie between the buildings, with some degree of enclosure provided by wings of buildings, trees, hedges, fences, arcades, or columned
walkways, become an entity with a positive quality (Alexander et al., 1977).
Courtyards in positive convex shapes are able to effectively extend the building boundaries, thereby providing more external views and connections to
therapeutic nature. Positive outdoor gardens and landscaping affordances
can become high activity areas; for instance, an exterior terrace/garden
adjacent to the dining court of a hospital is better utilized than any other
type of outdoor spaces on a medical campus, as proven by empirical observations (Jiang et al., 2018).

Patterns from Alexander et al. (1977):

- 69—Public outdoor room
- 105—South-facing outdoors
- 106—Positive outdoor space
- 115—Courtyards that live
- 176—Garden seat

Pattern 5: Micro-Landscapes along Narrow Wings

It has become desirable for natural ventilation and daylight to penetrate a
building envelope. Healthcare structures should be oriented to the natural
light as much as possible. Generally, buildings made up of long and narrow
wings reduce the depth of the interior space and enhance the exposure to
daylight, as seen in the building configuration of the Paimio Sanatorium
(1929–1933) by Alvar Aalto (see Chapter 4, Figure 4.3).

Patterns from Alexander et al. (1977):

- 95—Building complex
- 107—Wings of light
- 109—Long thin house
- 159—Light on two sides of every room

Pattern 6: Cascading Roof Terraces

Many memorable and beloved buildings throughout history have featured
cascading roofs, with projecting building elements, unfolding into a pro-
gression of smaller massing and roof elements. On the campus of a building
complex, flat roofs and terraces can be designed as gardens, especially if
limited lands on the ground level are allowed for therapeutic landscapes.
Roof gardens or terraces at various stories create a cascading greenery
that expands nature from the ground to the upper level of the building.

Cascading roof terraces could provide privacy and secure in the facility as an oasis in a high-density environment where at-grade resources are limited (Cooper-Marcus & Sachs, 2014).

Patterns from Alexander et al. (1977):

- 95—Building complex
- 108—Connected buildings
- 116—Cascade of roofs
- 118—Roof garden

Pattern 7: Transparent Arteries

Circulation arteries as the linkages between the functional units should be inviting and transparent, affording views of attractive landscapes throughout the diverse interior realms within a medical center campus. This pattern is also inspired by the "mover space" concept in the study of public spaces for healthcare facilities by Pangrazio (2013). Arteries feature constant movement as well as an ebb and flow of user volumes, including corridors and connecting bridges between different architectural components. Pasha (2013) found that gardens located in a hospital's low traffic zones are less likely to be discovered and used by visitors. In contrast, gardens located in a high traffic zone, such as at intersections or in central spaces (e.g., lobby or main corridor), are more likely to be passed by and discovered. Corridors, connecting bridges and walkways, indoor/outdoor walking tracks, and vertical circulation elements such as glass-sheathed elevators and escalators are essential to enhance the person–nature connection in the public areas of hospitals.

Patterns from Alexander et al. (1977):

- 31—Promenade
- 98—Circulation realms
- 101—Building thoroughfare
- 108—Connected buildings
- 119—Arcades
- 131—The Flow through rooms

Pattern 8: Landscaped Arrival Zones

The main arrival zones and emergency department entrances of a hospital are often abrupt, lacking inviting esthetic attributes to soften the transition into the monotonous institutional realm of the hospital. This pattern promotes the use of nature and landscaping to avoid disorienting, sudden, or jarring transitions from the outer world to the inner world of the medical center. Single-family dwellings traditionally have front porches, where one can be seen and see others coming and going. This ambiance is reinterpretable throughout the campus, originating with bright entry portals and the establishment of axiality through the use of landscaping.

Patterns from Alexander et al. (1977):

* 53—Main gateways
* 102— Family of entrances
* 110—Main entrance
* 112—Entrance transition
* 122—Building fronts
* 131—The Flow through rooms

Pattern 9: Dematerialized Edges

According to Verderber (2010), the exteriors and edge conditions of the minimalist modern hospital are often harsh and excessively institutional. In fact, the exterior multidimensional edges of a hospital building can be highly porous, gridded, tactile, transparent, layered, and textured compared to the mid to late 20th-century brutalist hospital exteriors and their edge conditions. The dematerialized building edges allow for far more openness, varied compositional massing, stepped floor levels, and user-friendly roofscapes not merely limited to the façade of the building. For example, one should be able to walk outdoors from the patient room onto a roof terrace, balcony, or ground-level garden (Verderber, 2010). As Alexander and colleagues (1977, p. 778) explained,

> If people cannot walk out from the building onto balconies and terraces which look toward the outdoor space around the building, then neither they themselves nor the people outside have any medium which helps them feel the building and the larger public world are intertwined.

Patterns from Alexander et al. (1977):

* 119—Arcades
* 122—Building fronts
* 124—Activity pockets
* 125—Stair seats
* 160—Building edge
* 166—Gallery surround
* 168—Connection to the earth

Pattern 10: Atrium Gardens and Lightwells

A central atrium is capable of drawing much-needed daylight, natural ventilation, and spatial diversity deep within the building interior. In extreme climates, sitting or walking outside may not be possible due to excessive heat and humidity or excessively cold temperatures whereas an atrium garden or lightwell that is vegetated functions year-round via a skylight or one equipped with an operable roof (Cooper-Marcus & Sachs, 2014; Jiang & Verderber, 2016). Winter gardens in extreme climates and vertical lightwells can feature a canopy of trees, ground plantings, seating, and water features as well as even possibly water walls and ponds (Ulrich, 1999).

Patterns from Alexander et al. (1977):

- 126—Something roughly in the middle
- 128—Indoor sunlight
- 135—Tapestry of light and dark
- 175—Greenhouse
- 194—Interior windows

Pattern 11: Sequestered Gardens

This pattern describes the intimate yet reserved relationship between a garden and the building interiors. The relationship between a garden and its adjacent interiors is complex and spatially multi-faceted: If a garden is too close to the public realm, people may not use it because it is not private enough; however, if it is too far from the public realm, then it also will not be used because it is too isolated (Alexander et al., 1977). A series of gardens should be placed in some kind of half-way position, side-by-side with the major spatial components or along the major circulation zones, in a position that is half-hidden from the public spaces and half-exposed.

Patterns from Alexander et al. (1977):

- 111—Half-hidden garden
- 127—Intimacy gradient
- 163—Outdoor room
- 193—Half-open wall

Pattern 12: Therapeutic Viewing Places

"Rooms without a view are like prisons for the people who have to stay in them" (Alexander et al., 1977, p. 890). People staying in a hospital for any length of time need to be able to refresh themselves by looking at a world different from the one they are in. In hospital waiting areas, therapeutic views to the external world are essential to the stressed patients and families. Bay windows, large windows with low sills and comfortable seating, or a glazed alcove with a high level of transparency that enable people to look onto outdoor nature are relaxing and therapeutic viewing places.

Patterns from Alexander et al. (1977):

- 134—Zen view
- 150—A place to wait
- 180—Window place
- 192—Windows overlooking life

Notes

1. A full discussion of this topic can be found in Jiang and Ersoy (2017). Phenomenal transparency and spatial continuity as an urban approach. In *Emerging complexity transparency and architecture*. Aristotle University of Thessaloniki, Faculty of Engineering–School of Architecture.
2. Shorthand record of a conversation in Plzen with Adolf Loos (1930). Retrieved from https://cargocollective.com/adolfloos/Muller-House-Czech-Rupublic
3. The preliminary pattern language of transparent spaces in hospitals was first formalized in Jiang's (2015) doctoral dissertation and refined in Jiang and Verderber's (2016) article entitled "Landscape Therapeutics and the Design of Salutogenic Hospitals: Recent research."

References

Addington, M., Kienzl, N., & Intrachooto, S. (2001). Mat buildings and the environment. In H. Sarkis (Ed.), *Le Corbusier's Venice Hospital*. Prestel.

Alberti, L. B. (1988). *On the art of building in ten books*. MIT Press.

Alexander, C., Ishikawa, S., Silverstein, M., Jacobson, M., Fiksdahl-King, I., & Angel, S. (1977). *A pattern language: Towns, buildings, construction*. Oxford University press.

Alexander, C. (1979). *The timeless way of building*. Oxford University press.

Allard, P. (2001). Bridge over Venice. In Sarkis, H. (Eds.). *Le Corbusier's Venice Hospital and the mat building revival*. Prestel.

Allison, D. (2007). Hospital as city: Employing urban design strategies for effective wayfinding. *Health Facilities Management, 20*(6), 61–65.

Cooper Marcus, C., & Sachs, N. A. (2014). *Therapeutic landscapes: An evidence-based approach to designing healing gardens and restorative outdoor spaces*. John Wiley & Sons.

Corbusier, L. (1929). *Le Corbusier & Pierre Jeanneret, oeuvre complète: 1946-1952 (Vol. 5)*. Publié par W. Boesiger aux Editions Girsberger.

Frampton, K. (2007). *Modern architecture: A critical history* (4th ed.). Thames & Hudson World of Art.

Hille, T. (2011). *Modern schools: A century of design for education*. John Wiley & Sons.

Hoesli, B. (1997a). Bernhard Hoesli commentary. In C. Rowe, R. Slutzky, & B. Hoesli (Eds.), *Transparency*. Birkhauser.

Hoesli, B. (1997b). Transparent form-organization as an instrument of design. In C. Rowe, R. Slutzky, & B. Hoesli (Eds.), *Transparency*. Birkhauser.

Jiang, S. (2015). Encouraging engagement with therapeutic landscapes: Using transparent spaces to optimize stress reduction in urban health facilities (Publication number 1495) [PhD dissertation, Clemson University]. *All Dissertations*. https://tigerprints.clemson.edu/all_dissertations/1495

Jiang, S., & Ersoy, U. (2017). Phenomenal transparency and spatial continuity as an urban approach. In *Emerging complexity transparency and architecture*. Aristotle University of Thessaloniki, Faculty of Engineering–School of Architecture.

Jiang, S., Staloch, K., & Kaljevic, S. (2018). Opportunities and barriers to using hospital gardens: Comparative post occupancy evaluations of healthcare landscape environments. *Journal of Therapeutic Horticulture, 28*(2), 23–56.

Jiang, S., & Verderber, S. (2016). Landscape therapeutics and the design of saluto-genic hospitals: Recent research. *World Health Design*, *8*(2), 40–51.

Kaplan, R., Kaplan, S., & Ryan, R. (1998). *With people in mind: Design and management of everyday nature*. Island Press.

Kepes, G. (1944). *The language of vision*. Paul Theobald.

Leatherbarrow, D. (2004). *Topographical stories: Studies in landscape and architecture*. University of Pennsylvania Press.

Leatherbarrow, D. (2005). *Space, spaces and spatiality*. Silpakorn University.

Le Corbusier, & Jeanneret, P. (1937). *Le Corbusier et Pierre Jeanneret, oeuvre compléte 1910–1929*. Éditions d Architecture.

Loftness, V., & Snyder, M. (2008). Chapter 8: Where windows become doors. In S. R. Kellert, H. H. Heerwagen, & M. L. Mador (Eds.), *Biophilic design: The theory, science, and practice of bringing buildings to life* (pp. 119–131). Hoboken, NJ: John Wiley & Sons, Inc.

Loose, A. (1930). Shorthand record of a conversation in Plzeň (Pilsen). Retrieved from Loose, A. (n.d.). *Muller House, Czech Rupublic*. https://cargocollective.com/adolfloos/Muller-House-Czech-Rupublic

Maciuika, J. V. (2000). Adolf Loos and the aphoristic style: Rhetorical practice in early twentieth-century design criticism. *Design Issues*, *16*(2), 75–86.

Naegele, D. J. (2001). Savoye space: The sensation of the object. *Harvard Design Magazine*, *15*, 4–13.

Neutra, R. J., & Marlin, W. (1989). *Nature near: Late essays of Richard Neutra*. Capra Press.

Oechslin, W. (1997). Transparency: The search for a reliable design method in accordance with the principles of modern architecture. In C. Rowe, & R. Slutzky (Eds.), *Transparency*. Birkhauser.

Pangrazio, J. R. (2013). All access: Planning public spaces for health care facilities. *Health Facilities Management*, *26*(3), 26–30.

Pasha, S. (2013). Barriers to garden visitation in children's hospitals. *HERD: Health Environments Research & Design Journal*, *6*(4), 76–96.

Psarra, S. (2012). A shapeless hospital, a floating theatre and an island with a hill: The invisible architecture of Venice. In *The proceedings to the eighth international space syntax symposium* (pp. K016–K016). Space Syntax Symposium.

Redfield, W. (2005). The suppressed site: Revealing the influence of site on two purist works. In C. J. Burns, & A. Kahn (Eds.), *Site matters: Design concepts, histories and strategies* (pp. 185–222). Routledge

Rowe, C., & Slutzky, R. (1963). Transparency: Literal and phenomenal. *Perspecta*, *8*, 45–54. doi:10.2307/1566901

Rowe, C., & Slutzky, R. (Eds.). (1997). *Transparency*. Birkhauser.

Rudofsky, B. (1969). *Streets for people: A primer for Americans*. Doubleday.

Samuel, F. (2010). *Le Corbusier and the architectural promenade*. De Gruyte.

Sarkis, H., Allard, P., & Hyde, T. (Eds.). (2001). *Le Corbusier's Venice Hospital and the Mat building revival*. Prestel Pub.

Schmarsow, A. (1993). The essence of architectural creation. In R. Vischer, C. Fiedler, H. Wolfflin, & A. Goller (Eds.), *Empathy, form and space—Problems in German aesthetics, 1873–1893* (pp. 125–148). Getty Center for the History of Art and the Humanities.

Setola, N., & Borgianni, S. (2016). *Designing public spaces in hospitals*. Routledge.

Shah, M. (2013). *Le Corbusier's Venice Hospital project: An investigation into its structural formulation*. Routledge.

Sitte, C. (1986). *City planning according to artistic principles*. Rizzoli.

Smithson, A. (1991). *Team 10 meeting 1953–1984*. Rizzoli.

Sternberg, E. M. (2009). *Healing spaces: The science of place and well-being*. Harvard University Press.

Tyson, M. M. (1998). *The healing landscape: Therapeutic outdoor environments*. McGraw-Hill.

Ulrich, R. S. (1999). Effects of gardens on health outcomes: Theory and research. In Cooper-Marcus, C., & Barnes, M. (Eds.), *Healing gardens: Therapeutic benefits and design recommendations*. John Wiley & Sons.

Verderber, S. (2010). *Innovations in hospital architecture*. Routledge.

Verderber, S., & Fine, D. J. (2000). *Healthcare architecture in an era of radical transformation*. Yale University Press.

Wright, F. L. (1955). In E. Kaufman (Ed.), *An American architecture*. Horizon Press.

6 The Effects of Windows and Transparency on People's Waiting Experience in Hospital Environments

Patients and their companions encounter waiting in almost every part of the healthcare journey—from the identification of a healthcare problem to its diagnosis and treatment and anticipation of a disease outcome (Fogarty & Cronin, 2008). The places where waiting happens, defined as healthcare waiting areas, are the first places where many patients experience mental and emotional activities; they are in-between places and "borderlands that face inwards to 'patienthood' and outwards to citizen status" (Clapton, 2018, p. 13). Waiting reflects people's helplessness and inability to control the pace of the healthcare process, which could lead to anxiety and stress, negative moods, and the feeling of having been forgotten (Clapton, 2018; Fux-Noy et al., 2019; Spechbach et al., 2019). The healthcare waiting experience is among the top-ranked issues in healthcare services, and the design of a supportive, positive healthcare waiting area is a continuing topic of concern for medical planners and healthcare architects.

Fogarty and Cronin (2008) conducted a concept analysis on patients' waiting experience for healthcare, with a focus on the period of time between the identification of a healthcare problem and its diagnosis and treatment, including the times spent on a waiting list. They identified the critical attributes of healthcare waiting: (1) period of measured time, (2) subjective interpretation of the perceived significance of the measured time, (3) feelings of uncertainty and powerlessness, and (4) anticipation of a response to the healthcare need (Fogarty & Cronin, 2008, p. 467). A body of research has investigated different patients' behaviors and experiences in different types of healthcare facilities, such as adults and children in general practice facilities (McDonald et al., 2020; Pati & Nanda, 2011), outpatient surgery facilities (Jafarifiroozabadi et al., 2021), mental health/psychotherapy facilities (Liddicoat, 2020; Noble & Devlin, 2021), oncology clinics (Blaschke et al., 2017), and emergency departments (EDs) (Ding et al., 2010; Nanda et al., 2012).

Waiting time could be substantially long in certain facilities, such as EDs: At the 90th percentile, patients experienced 105–222 minutes waiting time according to the 1-year visit data across four EDs in the United States while the acuity level 3 patients waited the longest time across all cases (Ding

DOI: 10.4324/9781003122180-6

et al., 2010). Despite the varied waiting times in different types of facilities, the waiting experience is commonly tedious and even stressful for many patients and their companions. Under the common goal of shortening (perceived) waiting time for healthcare and improving waiting experience, a study about healthcare waiting area design is documented in this chapter, followed by a series of evidence-based design implications as summarized from additional empirical studies on this topic.

Research Questions and Hypotheses

In this chapter, the pattern of "therapeutic viewing places" was explored based on people's perceptions of the design attributes of transparency in waiting areas in general healthcare environments.[1] In this study, it was hypothesized that the transparent healthcare waiting area was the most effective in reducing people's stress and calming their mood status compared to two other typical design typologies—namely, waiting areas with limited window views to nature and waiting areas with no window views to nature. Another hypothesis was that people preferred transparent healthcare waiting areas to other types of waiting areas in general healthcare environments.

The hypotheses were converted to following three groups of measurable research questions for this study:

- How do transparency design attributes in healthcare waiting areas affect people's mood status in such spaces? More specifically, what are people's mood scores after being exposed to three types of hospital waiting areas: (a) the total exclusion of nature, (b) limited window views to nature, or (c) transparent spaces with maximum natural views?
- How do transparency design attributes in healthcare waiting areas affect people's visual preferences for such spaces? More specifically, what are people's visual preference for three categories of images of hospital waiting areas: (a) the total exclusion of nature, (b) limited window views to nature, or (c) transparent spaces with maximum natural views?
- What additional factors contribute to the differences in visual preferences for the three categories of hospital waiting areas?

Research Design

The entire study consists of two phases. First, Study 1 was conducted through focus groups to select appropriate images that represent different levels of transparency in healthcare waiting area design. A survey-embedded quasi-experiment (Study 2) was then conducted in a lab to explore the impacts of different waiting areas on people's stress, mood, and visual preference. The waiting areas were simulated by projecting large-format images selected from Study 1. The two studies used different samples under different research design and methods.

Study 1: Image Selection

The purpose of Study 1 was to address the content validity issues in the study. "Content validity refers to the extent to which items represent the construct they are purported to measure" (Terry et al., 1999, p. 863). As "transparent healthcare waiting area" was a new construct, selecting the best representative images to ensure content validity was a prerequisite of the entire study. Similar to the methods used by Vincent (2009) and McNair et al. (2003), Study 1 adopted a mixture of methods in which both a sample of representative participants ($N = 19$) and a panel of experts ($N = 4$) reviewed, ranked, and selected the images of healthcare waiting areas to be used in Study 2, following a three-stage procedure. First, more than 100 images of waiting areas depicting general hospital or general clinical environments were sourced from multiple repositories, including professional design publications, design firms' websites, and open sources on the Internet. A set of criteria were then used to screen and narrow the primary selection to 54 images, with 18 images in each category of healthcare waiting areas design. The selection criteria are listed below (Jiang et al., 2017, pp. 53–54).

- Images depicting waiting rooms or waiting areas in the lobbies of general hospitals or general outpatient clinical environments were selected. To control variables, waiting areas in specialty healthcare facilities were eliminated, such as children's hospitals and EDs.
- Images were taken from the viewer's typical viewing angle and viewing position at the eye level.
- Images were kept consistent with the viewer's perception of the room spaciousness.
- Images were kept consistent with color themes.
- No obvious people were present in the images.

A small sample of participants ($N = 19$) were subsequently invited to participate in several focus group sessions and review the 54 images. In each session, participants were first introduced to the constructs of transparency and transparent spaces. They were then asked to sort the images into three categories of healthcare waiting area design: (a) the total exclusion of nature, (b) limited window views to nature, and (c) transparent spaces with maximum natural views. Finally, the participants were asked to rank the images within each category, from the most to the least representative of the category definition. They were told that it was not a preference survey, but to sort and rank the images according to their understanding of the constructs used in the study and the category definitions. A panel of experts ($N = 4$) reviewed the study results from the previous phase and provided extra comments to further guide the image selection. Finally, the top seven ranked images in each category were selected as the representatives of that particular category of healthcare waiting area design.

Study 2: The Survey-Embedded Quasi-Experiment

A survey-embedded, between-group, quasi-experiment was conducted to measure the mood-calming effects of different categories of healthcare waiting area designs. A total of 95 college students (males = 48, females = 47) were randomly recruited and purposefully matched to enroll in one of three study groups. Each participant was required to complete a series of demographic questions and remain calm in the lab for 5 minutes (i.e., pre-study calming period). Then each participant watched a thrilling 5-minute video that was purposefully selected to induce stress. Using a thriller movie as a stressor has been used in psychological studies (Thayler & Levenson, 1983; Ulrich et al., 1991; Wessel et al., 2008). Next, each participant watched a large image of the healthcare waiting area for 8 minutes while imaging they were in a healthcare waiting scenario (i.e., imagery treatment period). The top two ranked images for each category in Study 1 were used to represent each type of waiting area design; participants were randomly assigned to either of the two waiting area images within each study group. Both the stressor video and waiting area images were projected onto a large screen in the lab room. Right after the image-watching period, each participant was asked to complete the Profile of Mood States Survey Brief Form (POMS-Brief), a 30-item mood survey questionnaire (McNair et al., 2003). After the mood survey, each participant was invited to complete a preference survey to rate 21 images (i.e., a mixture of the three types of waiting area designs projected on the screen in random order), using a 6-point Likert scale. Prior to as well as during the stress video, each participant's heart rate and blood pressure were continuously measured using a medical grade vital monitor as indicators for the stress fluctuation. Figure 6.1 maps the study procedures of Study 2, and Figure 6.2 illustrates the images used in the imagery

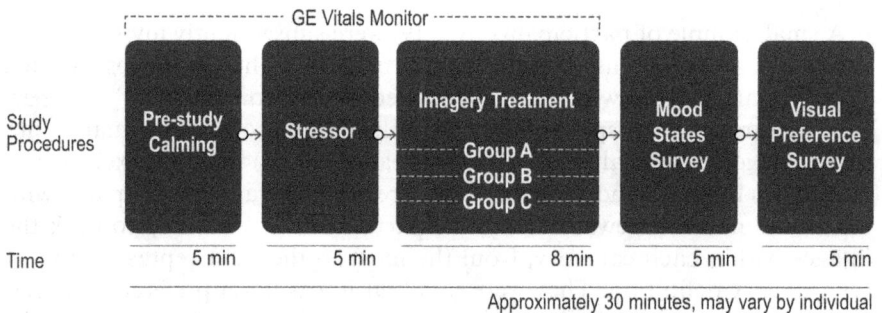

Figure 6.1 Study 2 research procedures. Group A = no window view; Group B = limited window view of nature; Group C = transparent space with maximum natural view

Source: Drawn by Shan Jiang

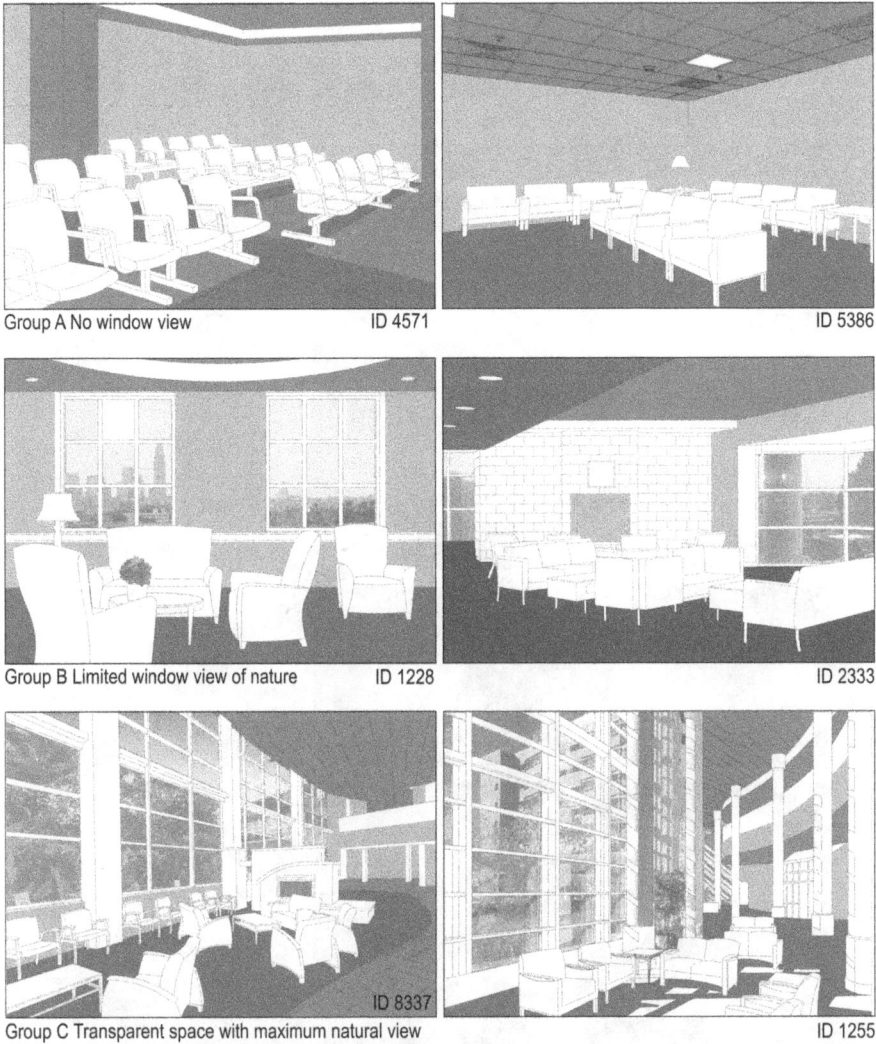

Group A No window view   ID 4571

ID 5386

Group B Limited window view of nature   ID 1228

ID 2333

Group C Transparent space with maximum natural view   ID 8337

ID 1255

Figure 6.2 The images[2] used in the imagery treatment period ($N = 6$)

Source: Drawn by Shan Jiang and Udday Datta

treatment period ($N = 6$) and Figure 6.3 illustrates the images used in the visual preference survey ($N = 21$).

Study 2 was conducted in the black-box room in the clinical simulation training lab at the School of Nursing at Clemson University, South Carolina. Comfortable seats with side tables were arranged in the center of the lab room (which was approximately 15 feet by 18 feet). Participants sat

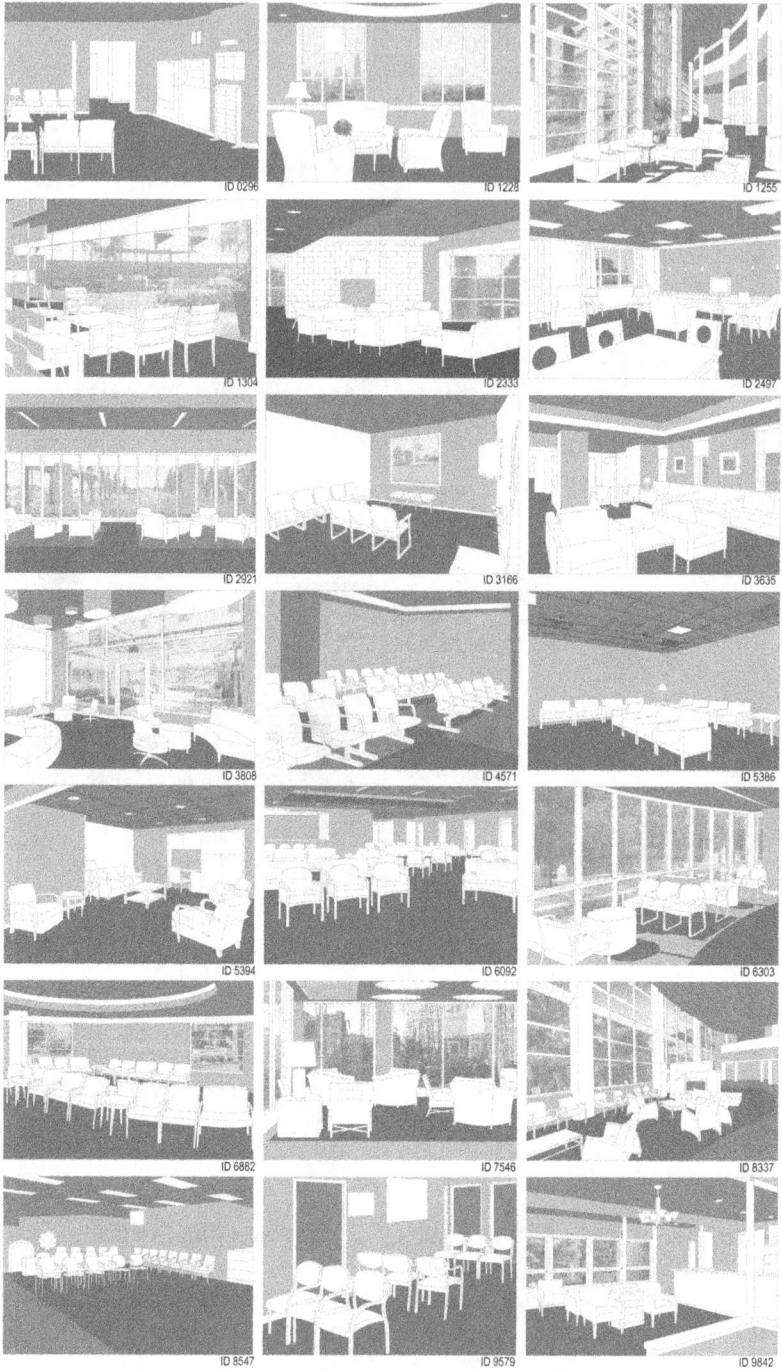

Figure 6.3 The images used in the visual preference survey ($N = 21$)

Source: Drawn by Shan Jiang and Udday Datta

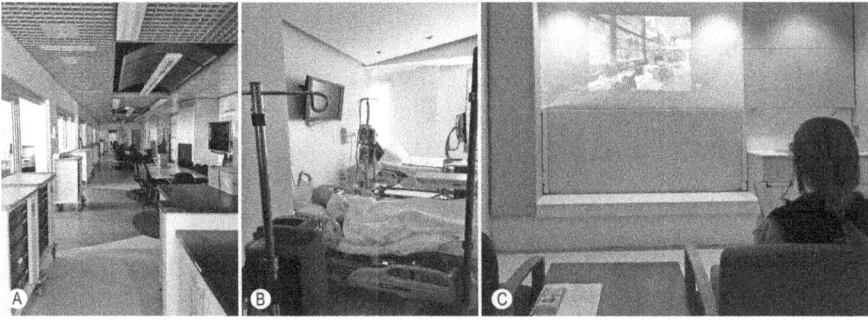

Figure 6.4 The clinical simulation training lab nurse stations (A), the simulated patient room (B), and the black-box room that was converted to a simulated waiting room (C) during study 2

Source: Photographer: Shan Jiang

in the chairs and faced a screen wall onto which the video and images were projected. A workspace was arranged behind the seats and participants to avoid distractions. Figure 6.4 depicts the lab room arrangement and the environmental context where the study was conducted.

Data Analysis and Results

Ninety-five participants' datasets were analyzed, including 48 males and 47 females. Eighty-nine participants were 18–30 years old, five participants were 31–45 years old, and one participant was above 60 years old. In addition, 63.2% of all participants ($N = 60$) were enrolled in a bachelor's degree program, 32.6% ($N = 31$) in a master's degree program, and 4.2% ($N = 4$) in a doctorate or postdoctoral level program. There were 31 participants (males = 17, females = 14) assigned to Group A, 34 participants (males = 15, females = 19) assigned to Group B, and 30 participants (males = 16, females = 14) assigned to Group C. The distribution of ethnicity among the three groups was consistent.

Stress-Inducing Effect of Watching a Movie Stressor

To test the healthcare waiting area designs' impacts on people's stress level and mood status in a lab setting, the research stimulated participants' stress level at the beginning of the study. Participants' heart rate as well as systolic and diastolic blood pressures was used as indicators of their perceived level of stress. The following formulas were used to process data:

Stress – Inducing Effect = (Xstress – Xpre) / Xpre × 100%

A one-sample t-test suggested significant ($p < .001$) differences occurred between the baseline values and the physiological readings during the stressor movie period. The average increase of all participants' systolic blood pressure was 4.0% (SD = 3.93), the average increase of diastolic blood pressure was 4.2% (SD = 5.57, p < .001), and the average increase of heart rate was 3.4% (SD = 5.90, p < .001). All analyses mentioned in this section suggest that the stressor demonstrated a significant stress-inducing effect.

Comparison of Psychophysiology Readings

To define the calming effect of different images in the three study groups, a formula was developed. The highest reading during the movie stressor was the most stressful status (X_{stress}), and the mean of the participant's post-movie-stressor readings was an indicator of the recovering period ($X_{recover}$); thus, the stress-reducing effect (by percentage) was defined as

$$Stress - Reducing\ Effect = (X stress - X_{recover}) / X_{pre} \times 100\%$$

The calming effect on systolic pressure suggested that the mean of participants' systolic pressure decreased 5.76% (SD = 4.33) while viewing the image in Group C and the decrease in Group B and Group A was 5.44% (SD = 3.37) and 5.33% (SD = 3.83), respectively. A one-way ANOVA analysis indicated the trend that Group C had the most stress-reducing effect compared to the other two treatment groups, $F(2, 93)$ = .103, p = .902, but the result was not statistically significant.

Comparison of Mood Scores

Reliability is the fundamental issue in psychological measurement (Ghiselli et al., 1981). Reliability includes two meanings: internal consistency, which is concerned with the homogeneity of the items comprising a scale (DeVellis, 1991), and the test–retest reliability, which refers to the stability of the questionnaires over time (Kline, 2000). The Cronbach's alpha coefficient is a widely accepted indicator of internal consistency (Cronbach, 1951). A scale with a very high Cronbach's alpha coefficient is unnecessary and may indicate redundancy in questionnaire items; a lower than .5 coefficient is considered very low reliability and unacceptable (George & Mallery, 2003). The POMS-Brief scale used in the study consists of six subscales; therefore, the internal consistency for each subscale was calculated. Five subscales' responses met the threshold and were reported; the confusion subscale was eliminated due to an unacceptable Cronbach's alpha coefficient.

A series of one-way ANOVAs with post-hoc paired comparisons were applied to the mean comparison of participants' tension, depression, anger, vigor, and fatigue scores. Statistically significant differences emerged among the three groups of participants, particularly on depression and anger sub-scales for female participants. Female participants from Group A reported a significantly higher depression score (N = 14, M = 1.93, SD = 2.43) than

Table 6.1 Multiple Comparisons of Depression and Anger Scores among Female
Participants

					90% Confidence interval	
(I) Group	*(J) Group*	*Mean difference (I-J)*	*Std. error*	*Sig.*	*Lower bound*	*Upper bound*
		Sum_Depression (Female); Test: LSD				
A	B	1.50752*	.53077	.007	.6157	2.3993
	C	1.71429*	.56957	.004	.7573	2.6713
B	A	−1.50752*	.53077	.007	−2.3993	−.6157
	C	.20677	.53077	.699	−.6851	1.0986
C	A	−1.71429*	.56957	.004	−2.6713	−.7573
	B	−.20677	.53077	.699	−1.0986	.6851
		Sum_Anger (Female); Test: LSD				
A	B	.59398*	.31465	.066	.0653	1.1227
	C	.71429*	.33764	.040	.1470	1.2816
B	A	−.59398*	.31465	.066	−1.1227	−.0653
	C	.12030	.31465	.704	−.4086	.6490
C	A	−.71429*	.33764	.040	−1.2816	−.1470
	B	−.12030	.31465	.704	−.6490	.4084

participants from Group B ($N = 19$, M = .42, SD = 1.02) and Group C ($N = 14$,
M = .21, SD = .58), $F(2, 44) = 5.584$, $p = .007$, significant at the .01 level.
Female participants from Group A also reported a marginally significant
higher anger score ($N = 14$, $M = .86$, $SD = 1.51$) than participants from Group
B ($N = 19$, M = .26, SD = .45) and Group C ($N = 14$, M = .14, SD = .36),
$F(2, 44) = 2.636$, $p = .083$, at the .1 significance level (Table 6.1).

Visual Preference Analysis

Comparison of Means

Each participant rated 21 images of hospital waiting areas based on their
individual visual preference using a 6-point Likert scale (1 = "extremely
dislike"; 6 = "extremely like"). The 21 images consisted of three categories
of hospital waiting areas, including hospital waiting rooms with window
views ($N = 7$), limited window views of nature ($N = 7$), and transparent space
with maximum views of nature ($N = 7$). A repeated measures ANOVA was
conducted to explore the differences among the three categories of images
regarding participants' visual preference scores. There was a significant main
effect of transparent waiting area with maximum natural views on participants' visual preference, Wilks' Lambda = .124, $F(2, 93) = 329.659$, $p < .001$.
Pairwise comparisons indicated significant differences in visual preference
for healthcare waiting areas without window views (category 1) ($M = 2.69$,

SD = .67), healthcare waiting areas with a limited window view of nature (category 2) (*M* = 3.60, *SD* = .57), and transparent healthcare waiting areas with a maximum natural view (category 3) (*M* = 4.88, *SD* = .55), *p* < .001.

Level of Transparency and Visual Preference

The relationship between people's preferences and level of transparency of the hospital waiting room images was further examined. To quantify the exploration using still images, the level of transparency was operationalized as the ratio between window views and the entire image. A matrix of the level of transparency of all images used in the preference study was calculated. As shown in Figure 6.5, the ratio of window views on all images from Category 1 was labeled as "0.0%" because of the lack of window views to nature. The ratios of window views to nature on images from Category 2 ranged from 1.6% to 21.4%. In Category 3, the images typically have full-sized window views to nature, and the ratios ranged from 34% to 46.7% (Jiang et al., 2017).

A Pearson correlation analysis was conducted on all participants' preference scores. A significant correlation exists between the preference scores and the level of transparency, which indicated that people's preference for healthcare waiting areas was related to the window size and the amount of natural views (*r* = .737, *p* < .001). In addition, a simple linear regression analysis of the preference data showed a significant positive linear correlation between the preference score (dependent variable) and the level of transparency (independent variable; *p* < .001), as shown in Figure 6.6.

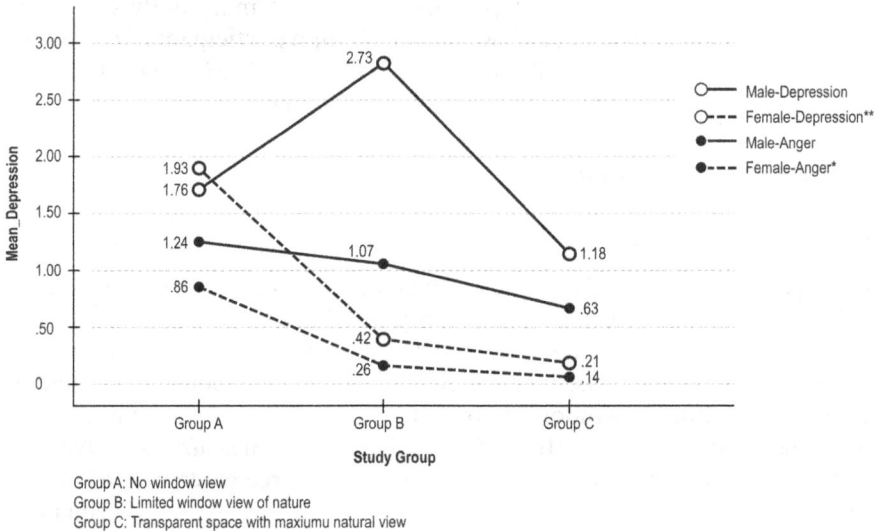

Group A: No window view
Group B: Limited window view of nature
Group C: Transparent space with maxiumu natural view

Figure 6.5 Between-group comparisons of participants' depression and anger scores by gender

Source: Drawn by Shan Jiang

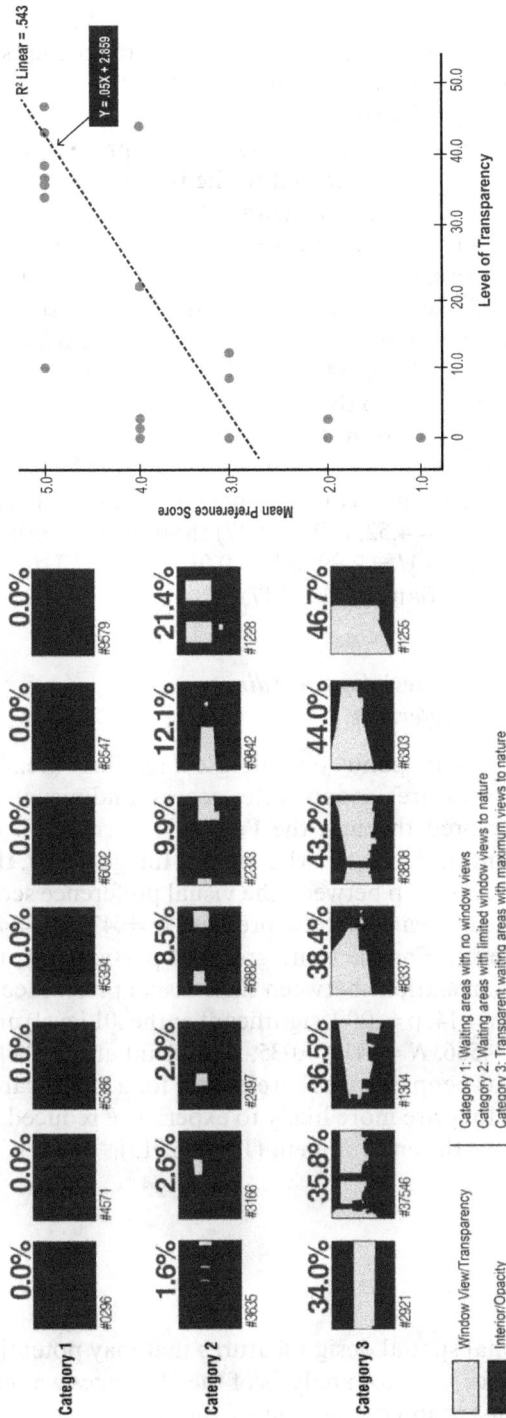

Figure 6.6 Level of transparency of healthcare waiting areas shown on the images in three categories (left) and the correlation between participants' preference scores and the levels of transparency of healthcare waiting areas (right)

Source: Drawn by Shan Jiang, originally published in Jiang et al. (2017, p. 56). Reuse permitted by the journal editor

Seat Arrangement and Visual Preference

The 21 images indicated two types of seating arrangements—namely, institutional and noninstitutional arrangement. For the institutional seat arrangement, the majority of seats are arranged along the interior walls or with their backs to the windows. When windows are present in such situations, people's lines of sights are oriented to the inside rather than looking outside. Seats are usually lined up or arranged in a row as seen in a rigid institutional environment, resulting in a lack of social interaction in the healthcare waiting environment. Eleven images used in the study included the institutional type of seating arrangement. In contrast, the noninstitutional seating arrangement facilitates socialization in the healthcare waiting environment. Seats are clustered in angles according to small groups, and people's views are oriented to the outside when windows are present in such situations. Ten images used in the study included the noninstitutional type of seating arrangement. The repeated measures ANOVA indicated that images with a noninstitutional arrangement gained significantly higher visual preference scores ($M = 4.52$, $SD = 0.047$) than images with an institutional seating arrangement ($M = 2.99$, $SD = 0.065$), Wilks' Lambda = .151, $F(1, 94) = 528.323$, $p < .001$ (Jiang et al., 2017).

Correlations among Psychophysiology Readings, Mood States, and Visual Preference

The correlation among participants' physiological readings (i.e., heart rate, systolic, and diastolic pressure), mood states scores, and visual preference scores was further explored through the Pearson's correlation coefficient analysis. For participants in Group C who viewed Image #8337, there was a marginally positive relationship between the visual preference score on that image and the decrease of their diastolic pressure ($r = .477$, $N = 14$, $p = .085$, at the .1 significance level). For the same group of participants, there were significantly negative correlations between their visual preference score and the tension ($r = -.668$, $N = 14$, $p = .009$, significant at the .01 level) and depression mood scores ($r = -.566$, $N = 14$, $p = .035$, significant at the .05 level). The results indicated that, as people's visual preference for a healthcare environment image increases, they are more likely to experience reduced stress and enhanced mood states in the environment (Jiang, 2015).

Factor Analysis

Six Factors

To explore the additional spatial design features that may potentially affect people's visual preference, a factor analysis of the 21 images was conducted, followed by a between-group comparison of the preference scores by the identified factors using a repeated measures ANOVA. The Kaiser–Meyer–Olkin (KMO) measure of sampling adequacy revealed that the sample was adequate for the factor analysis (0.710). The KMO statistic can vary between 0 and 1.0, and Kaiser (1974) recommended accepting values that are above .50. Furthermore, values between .5 and .7 are considered mediocre, values between .7 and .8 are considered good, values between .8 and .9 are considered great, and values above .9 are considered superb (Kaiser, 1974). The Bartlett's test of sphericity revealed that significant relationships existed between the variables ($p < .001$). Assuming the factors were not highly correlated with each other, the orthogonal solution and Varimax rotation method were used in the factor analysis. From the total variance explained matrix, factors loading .40 or above were identified, and the 21 images fell into six factors as described in Table 6.2.

Between-Group Comparison of Visual Preference Scores by Factors

A repeated measures ANOVA was then conducted to compare the differences among the six factors on participants' visual preference scores, which indicated significant differences, Wilks's Lambda = 0.076, $F(5, 90) = 219.455$, $p < .001$. The images in Factor 2 ($M = 4.89$, $SD = 0.62$), Factor 4 ($M = 5.05$, $SD = 0.75$), and Factor 5 ($M = 4.60$, $SD = 0.86$) were significantly preferred by people, $p < .001$. People somewhat liked the images in Factor 3 ($M = 3.81$, $SD = 0.70$) and somewhat disliked the images in Factor 6 ($M = 3.06$, $SD = 0.85$); the images in Factor 1 ($M = 2.34$, $SD = 0.69$) were the least preferred by student participants, $p < .001$.

Contribution to Existing Knowledge

In the quasi-experimental study, 95 participants were randomly assigned into three study groups of simulated healthcare waiting areas. The results suggested that all participants' psychophysiological readings (i.e., heart rate, diastolic and systolic pressures) significantly increased during the movie stressor period, suggesting that using a thrilling movie was effective in inducing people's stress level. During the imagery treatment period, participants in the simulated healthcare waiting areas with no window views reported the lowest reduction (by percentage) on systolic pressure, diastolic pressure, and heart rate compared to the other two groups, but the results did not reach the statistical significance level. Female participants in the no window group reported significantly higher mood scores on the depression and anger subscales, indicating that isolation from the outside in a healthcare waiting area may result in a negative impact on people's mood states. Females may experience a stronger emotional turbulence when under a stressful condition, such as in the hospital environment, and gender characteristics may play a role in moderating people's healthcare waiting experience.

Table 6.2 Factor Analysis Results for Healthcare Waiting Area Design (Jiang et al., 2017, pp. 57–59)

Factor	Image ID[3]	Loading
Factor 1: No window or limited window views with an institutional seating arrangement. Factor 1 included six images with no window view or limited window views to nature and an institutional seating arrangement. Images in this factor have no direct visual connections to the outside from within the waiting area. **Initial Eigenvalues:** 5.417; $M = 2.34$, $SD = .69$	#3166 #4571 #8547 #5386 #6882 #0296	.826 .783 .770 .617 .532 .420
Factor 2: Transparent space with maximum natural views. Factor 2 included four images of transparent spaces with maximum natural views. All images from this factor contained a full-sized window with abundant natural views, clear visual connections to the outside, and definite perception of the depth of the space. Images in this factor also indicated moderately high complexity and tasteful interior design. **Initial Eigenvalues:** 2.646; $M = 4.89$, $SD = .62$	#3808 #1304 #2921 #7546	.723 .691 .669 .543
Factor 3: No window or limited window views to nature with a noninstitutional furniture arrangement. Factor 3 included five images with no window or limited window views to nature and a noninstitutional furniture arrangement. Seats in the images of this factor were arranged according to the social grouping arrangement. Images in this factor showed domestic amenities, such as a lamp, curtains, and comfortable furniture and seats. **Initial Eigenvalues:** 1.719; $M = 3.81$, $SD = .70$	#2497 #5394 #3635 #9842 #1228	.796 .767 .551 .476 .451
Factor 4: Limited or maximum natural views with the presence of natural materials and a fireplace. Factor 4 included one image of transparent space with a maximum natural view and one image of a waiting area with limited window views of nature. In both images, salient natural materials (e.g., stone materials) and a fireplace are present. **Initial Eigenvalues:** 1.355; $M = 5.05$, $SD = .75$	#8337 #2333	.830 .789
Factor 5: Transparent space with maximum natural views, abundant natural light, and perceivable warmth. Factor 5 included two images of a transparent space with maximum natural views, abundant natural light, and perceivable warmth. **Initial Eigenvalues:** 1.202; $M = 4.60$, $SD = .86$	#6303 #1255	.654 .619
Factor 6: Institutional furniture arrangement in the least defensible space. Factor 6 included two images with an institutional furniture arrangement in the least defensible space. Images in this factor depict neutral spaces without window views to nature. Furthermore, more than three doors to other rooms can be perceived from the vantage point, which may indicate a least defensible space with a lack of privacy. **Initial Eigenvalues:** 1.023; $M = 3.06$, $SD = .85$	#6092 #9579	.828 .500

"Windows are more than openings in an exterior wall and must be considered for their size and proportion" (Shepley, 2006, p. 36). Previous studies have primarily focused on the types of views with insufficient attention on the size of windows and the amount of outside views in healthcare environments. In Ulrich's (1984) ground-breaking study, patients viewed the outside through a standard sized window (approximately 1.83 meters in height and 1.22 meters in width). Verderber (1986) conducted a study on person–nature transactions in healthcare environments and evaluated a series of spaces ranging from highly windowed to windowless. The study documented in this chapter extends beyond the concept of window space; transparent spaces and transparency design have been coined into the pattern of therapeutic viewing places in healthcare design. As Ulrich et al. (2008) suggested, large windows with natural views should be designed in not only patient rooms, but also in procedure spaces, treatment rooms, and waiting areas. The findings from this study are transferable to healthcare spaces wherever seating opportunities are present, including the public areas in the ED, pre- and post-clinical surgical rooms, consulting rooms for certain specialties, and lounge rooms for family members and medical staff.

The study findings echoed some existing theoretical frameworks beyond healthcare design and support the preference-based explanation of nature's affective benefits; people's spatial experience, mood, and affective responses in an environment could be mediated by their perception and preference over the environment (Herzog et al., 2003; Van den Berg et al., 2003; Wang et al., 2019). As hypothesized earlier by Loftness and Snyder (2008, p. 129), "the varying degrees of transparency" of a built environment influence each individual and the community regarding the extent of spiritual and affective status, and avoiding the sense of isolation and depression. Research findings from the current study have provided some direct evidence to support that windows and openings of a building should enable the occupants to access the richness of the outside world and connect humans and nature as much as possible.

Implications for Hospital Waiting Area Design

Waiting time should be shortened whenever possible for an optimal healthcare waiting experience. However, when waiting is inevitable, the design of the physical environment for waiting can make a significant difference in alleviating people's stress and support their emotional status. Waiting areas designed with transparency attributes are preferred by people dealing with stressful conditions in a simulated healthcare environment. Compared to the traditional window or no window conditions, healthcare waiting areas with the following transparency features may gain the optimum visual preference: (1) floor-to-ceiling windows or larger window–wall ratio with maximum views to the outside, (2) abundant views to the external therapeutic landscapes with high greenery ratio, and (3) bountiful natural light and perceivable warmth in a large space. Furniture arrangement patterns and interior design features may also enhance people's visual preference of the healthcare waiting area design. The noninstitutional furniture arrangement could promote interpersonal communication and social support; seats should cluster along the window in a social grouping pattern with a direct visual connection to the outside. The application of natural materials, such as wood and stone, and the presence of a fireplace add a domestic atmosphere and a sense of familiarity to the waiting area, making them preferred by people.

Beyond the scope of the study documented in this chapter, a literature review has been conducted on 45 empirical studies published since 2010 on topics of healthcare waiting experience and the relevant design issues. Preliminary findings are highly condensed through the following bullet points that fall into five themes, with the emphasis placed on the evidence-based design implications for future practices.

Spatial Layout, Amenities, and Aesthetics

- Large, spacious waiting rooms and welcoming features in psychotherapy offices are preferred (Noble & Devlin, 2021).
- Natural materials for the interior design, such as stone, brick, and wood decorations, are favorable attributes; home-like interior designs with comfortable seating, lamps, and a fireplace may induce the sense of relaxation and be more preferred by people (Jiang et al., 2017).
- Lighting conditions, space, ceiling height, and flooring style were additional environmental dimensions frequently mentioned by patients when discussing the design of a healthcare waiting area (Vuong et al., 2012).
- Alternative outdoor waiting spaces were preferred for sensory, cultural, social, and psychological reasons as an expression of the connectedness to kin and land by certain populations (O'Rourke et al., 2020).
- A coffee station is highly preferred (Noble & Devlin, 2021), and a play zone should be incorporated into the waiting area at pediatric or general practice facilities to keep the younger visitors occupied, thereby reducing adults' stress levels (Jiang, 2020; O'Rourke et al., 2020).

Positive Distractions

- Positive distractions in healthcare waiting areas that reduce patient anxiety and stress include views of nature, music, and visual art (Arneill & Devlin, 2002; Evans et al., 2009; Nanda et al., 2012; Pati & Nanda, 2011). Paintings depicting landscapes/nature scenes and animals/birds were highly preferred to abstract paintings or portraits (Cusack et al., 2010).
- The inclusion of nature features and nature-themed décor, such as plants, landscape art, and aquariums, in the waiting area at a variety

of healthcare facilities is highly preferred (Liddicoat, 2020; Noble & Devlin, 2021). Indoor plants and photos of plants work effectively in reducing patient stress in hospital waiting rooms (Baldwin, 2012), and artificial plants were rated better than no plants at all in an oncology clinic waiting room (Blaschke et al., 2017).

• Interactive media displays in a pediatric waiting space reduced waiting anxiety for children and their accompanying family members (Biddiss et al., 2013; Biddiss et al., 2014).

• Music interventions and aromatherapy could be effective distractions for adults in healthcare waiting areas (Biddiss et al., 2014; Fenko & Loock, 2014; Silverman, 2015). Nature sounds of ocean waves can reduce physiological and psychological stress as indicated by the muscle tension and pulse rate measurements in a healthcare waiting room environment (Largo-Wight et al., 2016).

• Cancer patients suggested organizing alternative activities, such as meeting with professionals and psychologists and engaging in fun activities (e.g., music therapy, drawing courses, library, TV programs) during the waiting period to enhance their emotional states (Catania et al., 2011).

Privacy, Support, and Control

• The provision of audial and visual privacy should be integrated into healthcare waiting area design (Jafarifiroozabadi et al., 2020; Liddicoat, 2020). The often conflicting demands for privacy and social interaction to support families and groups should be creatively addressed through design solutions (O'Rourke et al., 2020).

• The waiting room is a relational space and should be designed to provide social connectivity and opportunities for both children and adults to socialize in a pediatric waiting space (Corsano et al., 2015; Jiang, 2020).

• Patients' ability to control the environment (e.g., controlling lighting conditions through light levels and blinds) and time spent in the waiting areas should be maximized (Noble & Devlin, 2021).

• Cancer patients desire the control and freedom to leave the waiting room with a page and a personalized waiting experience during their waiting period (Catania et al., 2011).

Seating and Furniture

• A couch with armrests, a booth seat, and comfortable seats with soft textures were frequently preferred by people in the outpatient surgery waiting area. Being able to sit together was the top-ranked factor influencing seat selection among the patient and the care partner. The importance of factors, such as seat comfort, seat type, visual and auditory privacy, and the visibility to registration area, varied across different care task scenarios; however, the visual appearance of the seating remained equally important across all scenarios (Jafarifiroozabadi et al., 2020).

- Furnishings should suggest high quality (e.g., leather chairs), and softness and textiles should be included, such as throw pillows and blankets (Noble & Devlin, 2021).
- A range of sizes and types of seating as well as sufficient seating should be offered to increase variety and support privacy and choice. Distance between chairs should be provided to maintain privacy, and groupings of tables and chairs should be created to support families and patients with care providers (Noble & Devlin, 2021).
- Seats should be clustered along the window in a social grouping arrangement with direct visual connection to the outside (Jiang et al., 2017); a seating arrangement in the sense of homeyness improves the domestic feeling of the healthcare waiting space (Becker & Douglass, 2008).

Health Information and Resources

- Available health information, resources, and supports provided in the hospital waiting areas are infrequently and briefly accessed by occupants, among which the audiovisual displays were more frequently used than hardcopy items; it could be a trend to share digitalized health information within the waiting and clinical areas of healthcare facilities (McDonald et al., 2020).
- In the waiting areas at mental health facilities, the signage and labeling of the mental health service can exacerbate negative stigmas in the waiting area of a mental health facility; therefore, they should be carefully considered. The visible presence of security features increases people's feelings of otherness and difference and should be minimized wherever possible in the mental health facility (Liddicoat, 2020).
- A technology-based integrative medicine app to deliver guided acupressure and mindfulness meditation could significantly reduce patient stress, anxiety, and pain in a chemotherapy waiting room (Bao et al., 2019; Beukeboom et al., 2012).
- Audiovisual aids broadcasting messages using screens may enhance patients' knowledge of healthcare (Berkhout et al., 2018). Passive interventions of healthcare information in healthcare waiting areas had a general positive influence on promoting healthy lifestyle behaviors (Cass et al., 2016).
- A technology-based information screen intended to improve the perception of queuing and waiting time resulted in a high satisfaction rate related to the patient experience (Ehrler et al., 2016).
- Healthcare waiting areas have strong potentials to be redesigned to enhance families' engagement in and connection to community resources (Henize et al., 2018).

Notes

1. A peer-reviewed journal article related to this study can be found in *Health Environments Research & Design Journal* (Jiang et al., 2017).
2. The images originally used in the study were real photos with different degrees of manipulation aimed to fulfill the experiment requirement. The images were further converted into the diagrammatic style for this book due to copyright considerations.
3. Refer to Figure 6.3 for the ID information for each image.

References

Arneill, A. B., & Devlin, A. S. (2002). Perceived quality of care: The influence of the waiting room environment. *Journal of Environmental Psychology*, *22*(4), 345–360.

Baldwin, A. L. (2012). How do plants in hospital waiting rooms reduce patient stress? *The Journal of Alternative and Complementary Medicine*, *18*(4), 1–2.

Bao, T., Deng, G., DeMarzo, L. A., Zhi, W. I., DeRito, J. L., Blinder, V., Chen, C., Li, Q. S., Green, J., Pendleton, E., & Mao, J. J. (2019). A technology-assisted, brief mind–body intervention to improve the waiting room experience for chemotherapy patients: Randomized quality improvement study. *JMIR Cancer*, *5*(2), e13217.

Becker, F., & Douglass, S. (2008). The ecology of the patient visit: Physical attractiveness, waiting times, and perceived quality of care. *The Journal of Ambulatory Care Management*, *31*(2), 128–141.

Berkhout, C., Zgorska-Meynard-Moussa, S., Willefert-Bouche, A., Favre, J., Peremans, L., & Van Royen, P. (2018). Audiovisual aids in primary healthcare settings' waiting rooms. A systematic review. *European Journal of General Practice*, *24*(1), 202–210.

Beukeboom, C. J., Langeveld, D., & Tanja-Dijkstra, K. (2012). Stress-reducing effects of real and artificial nature in a hospital waiting room. *The Journal of Alternative and Complementary Medicine*, *18*(4), 329–333.

Biddiss, E., Knibbe, T. J., & McPherson, A. (2014). The effectiveness of interventions aimed at reducing anxiety in health care waiting spaces: A systematic review of randomized and nonrandomized trials. *Anesthesia & Analgesia*, *119*(2), 433–448.

Biddiss, E., McPherson, A., Shea, G., & McKeever, P. (2013). The design and testing of interactive hospital spaces to meet the needs of waiting children. *Health Environments Research & Design Journal*, *6*(3), 49–68.

Blaschke, S., O'Callaghan, C. C., & Schofield, P. (2017). "Artificial but better than nothing": The greening of an oncology clinic waiting room. *Health Environments Research & Design Journal*, *10*(3), 51–60.

Cass, S. J., Ball, L. E., & Leveritt, M. D. (2016). Passive interventions in primary healthcare waiting rooms are effective in promoting healthy lifestyle behaviours: An integrative review. *Australian Journal of Primary Health*, *22*(3), 198–210.

Catania, C., De Pas, T., Minchella, I., De Braud, F., Micheli, D., Adamoli, L., Spitaleri, G., Noberasco, C., Milani, A., Zampino, M. G., Toffalorio, F., Radice, D., Goldhirsch, A., & Nolè, F. (2011). "Waiting and the waiting room: How do you experience them?" Emotional implications and suggestions from patients with cancer. *Journal of Cancer Education*, *26*(2), 388–394.

Clapton, G. (2018, November). The general practice health waiting area in images: Threshold, borderland, and place of transition in the sense of self. *Forum Qualitative Sozialforschung/Forum: Qualitative Social Research, 19*(1). https://www.qualitative-research.net/index.php/fqs/article/view/2896/4175

Corsano, P., Majorano, M., Vignola, V., Guidotti, L., & Izzi, G. (2015). The waiting room as a relational space: Young patients and their families' experience in a day hospital. *Child: Care, Health and Development, 41*(6), 1066–1073.

Cronbach, L. J. (1951). Coefficient alpha and the internal structure of tests. *Psychometrika, 16*(3), 297–334.

Cusack, P., Lankston, L., & Isles, C. (2010). Impact of visual art in patient waiting rooms: Survey of patients attending a transplant clinic in Dumfries. *JRSM Short Reports, 1*(6), 1–5

DeVellis, R. F. (1991). *Scale development: Theory and applications (vol. 26).* Sage.

Ding, R., McCarthy, M. L., Desmond, J. S., Lee, J. S., Aronsky, D., & Zeger, S. L. (2010). Characterizing waiting room time, treatment time, and boarding time in the emergency department using quantile regression. *Academic Emergency Medicine, 17*(8), 813–823.

Ehrler, F., Siebert, J., Wipfli, R., Duret, C., Gervaix, A., & Lovis, C. (2016). Improving patients experience in paediatric emergency waiting room. *Studies in Health Technology and Informatics, 225*, 535–539.

Evans, J. D., Crooks, V. A., & Kingsbury, P. T. (2009). Theoretical injections: On the therapeutic aesthetics of medical spaces. *Social Science & Medicine, 69*(5), 716–721.

Fenko, A., & Loock, C. (2014). The influence of ambient scent and music on patients' anxiety in a waiting room of a plastic surgeon. *Health Environments Research & Design Journal, 7*(3), 38–59.

Fogarty, C., & Cronin, P. (2008). Waiting for healthcare: A concept analysis. *Journal of Advanced Nursing, 61*, 463–471.

Fux-Noy, A., Zohar, M., Herzog, K., Shmueli, A., Halperson, E., Moskovitz, M., & Ram, D. (2019). The effect of the waiting room's environment on level of anxiety experienced by children prior to dental treatment: A case control study. *BMC Oral Health, 19*(1), 1–6.

George, D., & Mallery, P. (2003). *SPSS for windows step by step: A simple guide and reference.* 11.0 update (4th ed.). Allyn & Bacon.

Ghiselli, E. E., Campbell, J. P., & Zedeck, S. (1981). *Measurement theory for the behavioral sciences: Origin & evolution.* WH Freeman & Company.

Henize, A. W., Beck, A. F., Klein, M. D., Morehous, J., & Kahn, R. S. (2018). Transformation of a pediatric primary care waiting room: Creating a bridge to community resources. *Maternal and Child Health Journal, 22*(6), 779–785.

Herzog, T. R., Maguire, P., & Nebel, M. B. (2003). Assessing the restorative components of environments. *Journal of Environmental Psychology, 23*(2), 159–170.

Jafarifiroozabadi, R., Joseph, A., Joshi, R., & Wingler, D. (2020). Evaluating care partner preferences for seating in an outpatient surgery waiting area using virtual reality. *Health Environments Research & Design Journal*, 1937586720922194.

Jiang, S. (2015). Encouraging engagement with therapeutic landscapes: Using transparent spaces to optimize stress reduction in urban health facilities [Doctoral dissertation]. *All Dissertations.* 1495. https://tigerprints.clemson.edu/all_dissertations/1495

Jiang, S. (2020). Positive distractions and play in the public spaces of pediatric healthcare environments: A literature review. *Health Environments Research & Design Journal, 13*(3), 171–197.

Jiang, S., Powers, M., Allison, D., & Vincent, E. (2017). Informing healthcare waiting area design using transparency attributes: A comparative preference study. *Health Environments Research & Design Journal, 10*(4), 49–63.

Kaiser, H. (1974). An index of factorial simplicity. *Psychometrika, 39*, 31–36.

Kline, P. (2000). *Handbook of psychological testing* (2nd ed.). Routledge.

Largo-Wight, E., O'Hara, B. K., & Chen, W. W. (2016). The efficacy of a brief nature sound intervention on muscle tension, pulse rate, and self-reported stress: Nature contact micro-break in an office or waiting room. *Health Environments Research & Design Journal, 10*(1), 45–51.

Liddicoat, S. (2020). The therapeutic waiting room: Therapist and service user perspectives on the psychologically supportive dimensions of architectural space. *Health Environments Research & Design Journal, 13*(2), 103–118.

Loftness, V., & Snyder, M. (2008). Chapter 8: Where windows become doors. In S. R. Kellert, H. H. Heerwagen, & M. L. Mador (Eds.), *Biophilic design: The theory, science, and practice of bringing buildings to life* (pp. 119–131). Hoboken, NJ: John Wiley & Sons, Inc.

McDonald, C. E., Remedios, L. J., Said, C. M., & Granger, C. L. (2020). Health literacy in hospital outpatient waiting areas: An observational study of what is available to and accessed by consumers. *Health Environments Research & Design Journal*, 1937586720954541.

McNair, D. M., Lorr, J., & Droppleman, L. F. (2003). *POMS brief form*. Multi-Health Systems Inc.

Nanda, U., Chanaud, C., Nelson, M., Zhu, X., Bajema, R., & Jansen, B. H. (2012). Impact of visual art on patient behavior in the emergency department waiting room. *The Journal of Emergency Medicine, 43*(1), 172–181.

Noble, L., & Devlin, A. S. (2021). Perceptions of psychotherapy waiting rooms: Design recommendations. *Health Environments Research & Design Journal*, 19375867211001885.

O'Rourke, T., Nash, D., Haynes, M., Burgess, M., & Memmott, P. (2020). Cross-cultural design and healthcare waiting rooms for Indigenous people in regional Australia. *Environment and Behavior*, 0013916520952443.

Pati, D., & Nanda, U. (2011). Influence of positive distractions on children in two clinic waiting areas. *Health Environments Research & Design, 4*, 124–140.

Shepley, M. M. (2006). The role of positive distraction in neonatal intensive care unit settings. *Journal of Perinatology, 26*, 34–37.

Silverman, M. J. (2015). Effects of live music in oncology waiting rooms: Two mixed methods pilot studies. *International Journal, 3*(1), 1–15.

Spechbach, H., Rochat, J., Gaspoz, J. M., Lovis, C., & Ehrler, F. (2019). Patients' time perception in the waiting room of an ambulatory emergency unit: A cross-sectional study. *BMC Emergency Medicine, 19*(1), 1–10.

Terry, P. C., Lane, A. M., Lane, H. J., & Keohane, L. (1999). Development and validation of a mood measure for adolescents. *Journal of Sports Sciences, 17*, 861–872.

Thayler, J. F., & Levenson, R. W. (1983). Effects of music on psychophysiological responses to a stressful film. *Psychomusicology: A Journal of Research in Music Cognition, 3*(1), 44.

Ulrich, R. S. (1984). View through a window may influence recovery from surgery. *Science, 224*(4647), 420–421.

Ulrich, R. S., Simons, R. F., Losito, B. D., Fiorito, E., Miles, M. A., & Zelson, M. (1991). Stress recovery during exposure to natural and urban environments. *Journal of Environmental Psychology, 11*(3), 201–230.

Ulrich, R. S., Zimring, C., Zhu, X., DuBose, J., Seo, H. B., Choi, Y. S., & Joseph, A. (2008). A review of the research literature on evidence-based healthcare design. *Health Environments Research & Design Journal, 1*(3), 61–125.

Van den Berg, A. E., Koole, S. L., & van der Wulp, N. Y. (2003). Environmental preference and restoration: (How) are they related? *Journal of Environmental Psychology, 23*(2), 135–146.

Verderber, S. (1986). Dimensions of person-window transactions in the hospital environment. *Environment and Behavior, 18*(4), 450–466.

Vincent, E. (2009). Therapeutic benefits of nature images on health [Doctoral dissertation]. *All Dissertations.* 432. https://tigerprints.clemson.edu/all_dissertations/432

Vuong, K. A., Cain, R., Burton, E., & Jennings, P. (2012). The impact of healthcare waiting environment design on end-user perception and well-being. *Environment, 3,* 6.

Wang, R., Zhao, J., Meitner, M. J., Hu, Y., & Xu, X. (2019). Characteristics of urban green spaces in relation to aesthetic preference and stress recovery. *Urban Forestry & Urban Greening, 41,* 6–13.

Wessel, I., Overwijk, S., Verwoerd, J., & de Vrieze, N. (2008). Pre-stressor cognitive control is related to intrusive cognition of a stressful film. *Behaviour Research and Therapy, 46*(4), 496–513.

7 The Effects of Windows and Transparency on People's Wayfinding Behaviors and Navigational Experience in Hospitals

Large Hospitals and the Wayfinding Issues

Large healthcare institutions are highly compartmentalized entities, with countless layers of functional requirements regulating their spatial attributes. Numerous support functions have been connected via a complicated network of internal and external circulation paths. As the facilities evolved through years of practices, the functional units and circulation spaces were shaped over time by the advanced medical technology and building techniques, resulting in maze-like environments and significant wayfinding issues in current large hospitals (Jiang & Verderber, 2017). As summarized by Cooper (2010), a combination of factors accelerates the spatial disorientation and wayfinding difficulties; the constant expansion and restructuring of the facilities usually result in differences in the design, scale, and orientation between the original building and the new additions. For inexperienced visitors, changing terminology, new procedures, and unexplained protocols usually cause confusion in hospital wayfinding. Elevators and entrances with restricted access for the purposes of security or infection control may unexpectedly cut the flow of individuals' cognitive mapping and make them feel totally lost (Cooper, 2010; Jiang, in progress). Research has reported that nearly one-third of first-time visitors to hospitals feel lost while approximately one out of every four hospital workers is confused about the locations of some critical destinations in the hospital (Medelita, 2017).

Hospital wayfinding issues could lead to late arrivals or missed appointments, unpleasant navigational experiences, and stress and anxiety. People's capability of processing the environmental information decreases in a stressful situation or under time pressure. The chaotic hospital environments compounding patients' sickly conditions could further intensify their stress and make patients and visitors feel lost more frequently. Indeed, in a survey study involving 247 staff from 12 hospitals, 52% of staff reported that they were asked for directions more frequently when the site was busy (Miller & Lewis, 2000). A good navigational experience in healthcare facilities could promote healing by providing patients and visitors with a sense of control, reduced stress, and enhanced emotional status, which could otherwise

DOI: 10.4324/9781003122180-7

undermine the body's immune system (Carpman et al., 1985). Healthcare providers have also identified wayfinding as a major factor related to the quality of their physical work environment that affects work efficiency and job satisfaction (Mourshed & Zhao, 2012). Improving hospital wayfinding could substantially reduce the financial burden to any healthcare system as Zimring (1990) revealed that the hidden costs of direction giving by staff members at a university hospital were equivalent to more than 4,500 staff hours.

In the guiding research report published by The Center for Health Design, "reducing spatial disorientation" was identified as one of the nine dimensions of environmental measures to improve patient outcomes in the 21st century (Ulrich et al., 2008). Public spaces in hospitals, including the circulation spaces and corridors, can promote memorable and positive experiences and contribute to the overall healing process through the provision of well-designed spatial orientation cues (Pangrazio, 2013). Jiang and Verderber (2017) summarized the vital roles that circulation spaces play in current hospital environments, including (1) the delivery of fundamental healthcare services, (2) essential components of patients' total healthcare experience, and (3) transitional linkages connecting interior spaces with the outside nature. Therefore, healthcare circulation spaces deserve adequate research and design attention equivalent to other spaces in hospital environments.

Certain urban design strategies may contribute to an efficient wayfinding system in healthcare design. As early as the 1960s, Lynch (1960) examined how people process environmental information and the relevant wayfinding issues in urban environments based on mental mapping. Five elements— paths, edges, districts, nodes, and landmarks—comprise the patterns of recognizable symbols in a legible city (Lynch, 1960). Hospitals are analogical to a small city due to the similarities in functional complexity. As suggested by David Allison (2007, p. 61), the leading influencer and educator in healthcare architecture, "hospitals, like cities, should have landmarks, public places and greenspaces for both therapeutic and navigational purposes." Carthey (2008) supported Allison's perspective, concluding that every corridor should "be considered a part of the larger circulatory system of a hospital, in much the same way urban streets are part of a hierarchy of connecting routes within a city" (p. 24). Designing the "main streets" with transparency attributes, known as transparent arteries, could link the various functional units with atrium gardens and lightwells, breathable courtyards, and extensive views to the outside, forming a promising internal structure that enhances the legibility and imageability of the hospital. In fact, previous studies on complex building configurations have indicated that strong visual connections/transparency to the destination facilitates navigators' spatial orientation and wayfinding (Carpman et al., 1985; Seidel, 1982). Buildings organized around an open core or a central atrium have the advantage of providing visual access to the form of the entire circulation system, thereby improving navigators' wayfinding performances (Arthur & Passini, 1992; Dogu & Erkip, 2000). Healthcare environments featuring abundant natural daylight in the circulation spaces support wayfinding and provide an inviting ambiance (Topo et al., 2012). In contrast, long and windowless corridors can be frightening and cause anxiety for new patients, "especially those who are not sure how far it might be and whether help is nearby" (Foureur et al., 2010, p. 49).

Research Questions and Hypotheses

To fill some significant research gaps in the field, as well as provide research evidence in support of the pattern transparent arteries, this chapter documents a recent study on the effects of windows and transparency on people's wayfinding behaviors and navigational experience in hospitals[1]. The study was based on two hypotheses—namely, having sufficient views to nature and daylight from within hospital circulation spaces could (1) facilitate people's wayfinding and spatial orientation and (2) enhance people's mood states and improve their spatial experience associated with wayfinding. The hypotheses were further translated into a series of specific research questions:

Comparing two types of hospital circulation spaces—(a) transparent spaces with sufficient window views of nature and daylight and (b) windowless corridors:

1 How do participants perform and behave differently regarding wayfinding in the two types of environments?
2 How do participants' mood states associated with wayfinding vary in the two types of environments?
3 What are the differences of participants' preferences to the environmental characteristics and atmosphere in the two types of environments?
4 What roles can the hospital gardens and nature views play during participants' wayfinding in the two types of environments?

Research Design

Experiment Setup

A controlled experiment was conducted on a total of 74 participants, with the survey and interview components integrated in the research design. Participants were randomly recruited and randomly assigned to either the nature group (i.e., Group A - transparent hospital circulation spaces that provide sufficient views to nature and daylight) or the control group (i.e., Group B - windowless corridors) to complete five wayfinding tasks within a limited time frame. Several aspects were compared between the two study groups, including participants' wayfinding performances and behaviors, their stress levels and mood states, and the preference to the environmental characteristics and atmosphere. The two types of hospital environments were constructed using computer modeling programs and delivered to the participants via the immersive virtual environment (IVE) techniques, also known as virtual reality (VR) techniques. Two IVEs were used to construct the typical comprehensive diagnostic and treatment hospital environment: a generous entry lobby, semi-restrictive prep/recovery area, treatment area, radiology unit, labs, and staff support area, all connected by interdepartmental corridors. Previous studies have indicated that people pay particular attention to the changes in the local geometry of the environments during wayfinding, such as corners, openings, and occlusions (Wiener et al., 2012). Therefore, four gardens were strategically placed at the key decision points in the IVE hospital for the nature group, in which participants could perceive continuous natural views as provided by the curtain walls along the gardens and the periphery of the building. In contrast, in the control group, the circulation spaces of the IVE hospital were constructed by solid walls without any window views to the outside. In other respects, the two groups shared an almost identical spatial layout and room arrangement as well as interior design and decorations.

The fully immersive VR experiences were delivered through HTC Vive Head Mounted Display (HMD) and SteamVR system. A room-scale experimental zone (approximately 6 foot by 8 foot clearance) in a lab was virtually defined through two base stations installed diagonally in the space. Participants wore a threaded HMD and were allowed to physically move and turn within the experimental zone while controlling the remote controller and navigating the designated IVE hospital. The navigation mode was preset as "walkthrough"; therefore, participants were able to "walk" in the continuous traveling mode in the IVE hospital. The researcher was able to observe each participant's wayfinding behaviors and record the entire navigation process using screen-recording software on the lab computers (Jiang, in progress).

Measurements and Data Collection Procedures

The experiment included five phases coordinated either before or after the IVE wayfinding tasks. As indicated in the flow chart in Figure 7.1, participants were oriented to the study procedures and consented to participate; their demographic information was then collected in the Pre-Experiment Preparation phase. Participants were then asked to view the floor map of the IVE hospital and get familiar with the space for two minutes before wearing the HMD because, once the wayfinding tasks started, they would no longer have access to the hospital floor map. They were trained to use the IVE goggles and remote controller to navigate the entry lobby of the IVE hospital as a warm-up practice. In the IVE Wayfinding Tasks phase, participants were asked to complete five wayfinding tasks within a 15-minute period;

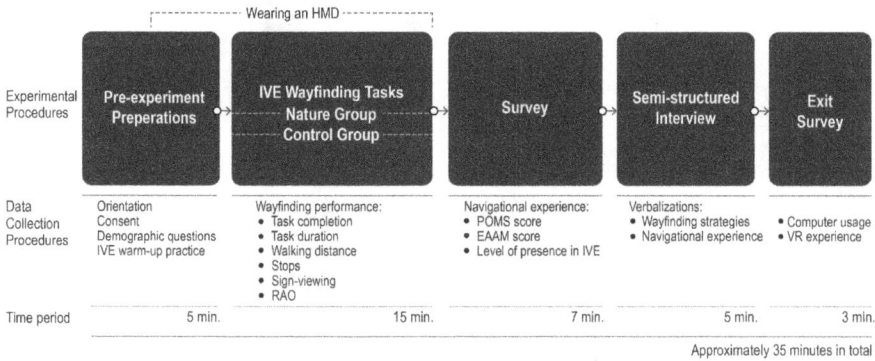

Figure 7.1 Research procedures. Nature group = transparent hospital circulation spaces that provide sufficient views to nature and daylight; control group = windowless corridors in the hospital

Source: Drawn by Shan Jiang

the tasks and optimal route for each task (defined by the shortest walking distance) are mapped in Figure 7.2. The tasks simulated a real-world situation in which patients "traveled" among different departmental units, including exam rooms, the radiology unit, and the lab. For both study groups, each room in the IVE had an exclusive room tag with a four-digit numerical room label, and basic ceiling signs were available to indicate the departmental units shown on the floor maps. No additional arrows, color coding, or visual cues were included in either IVE. Figure 7.3A–C depicts the real-time rendering of the IVE hospital as experienced by participants, taking the nature group as an example.

Participants then entered the Survey phase, when they completed several questionnaires that measured their mood states, the level of attractiveness and atmosphere perceived by participants, and the level of presence in the IVE hospitals. Three questionnaires were utilized in the Survey phase of the study. Immediately after the wayfinding tasks, each participant first completed the abbreviated version (30-item) of Profile of Mood States Survey (POMS-Brief) (McNair et al., 2003). POMS-Brief measures six domains of mood states, including tension, depression, anger, fatigue, confusion, and vigor; each domain consists of five questionnaire items that describe the degree of feeling that people have, using a 5-point Likert scale (0 = not at all; 4 = extremely). Then each participant took the Environmental Attractiveness and Atmosphere Metrics (EAAM), which consists of 20-item bipolar statements adapted from Vogels' (2008) study that measured the perceived level of esthetics and atmosphere of the IVE hospital environment based on a preference scale (i.e., 1 = ugly; 5 = attractive). Third, each participant took the 12-item IGroup Presence Questionnaire (IPQ), a questionnaire intended to measure people's level of presence and perceived level of reality in a virtual

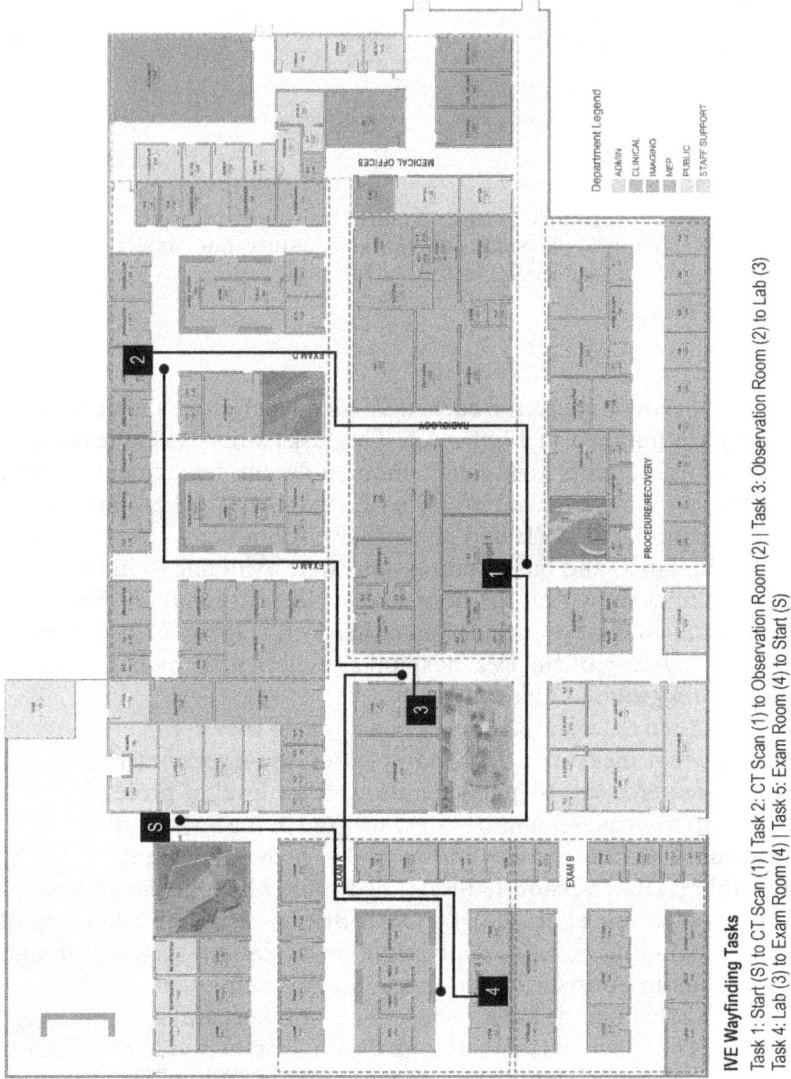

Figure 7.2 IVE wayfinding tasks and the optimal route for each task as defined by the shortest walking distance using the nature group situation for demonstration. The wayfinding tasks were the same for both the nature and control groups

Source: Drawn by Shan Jiang

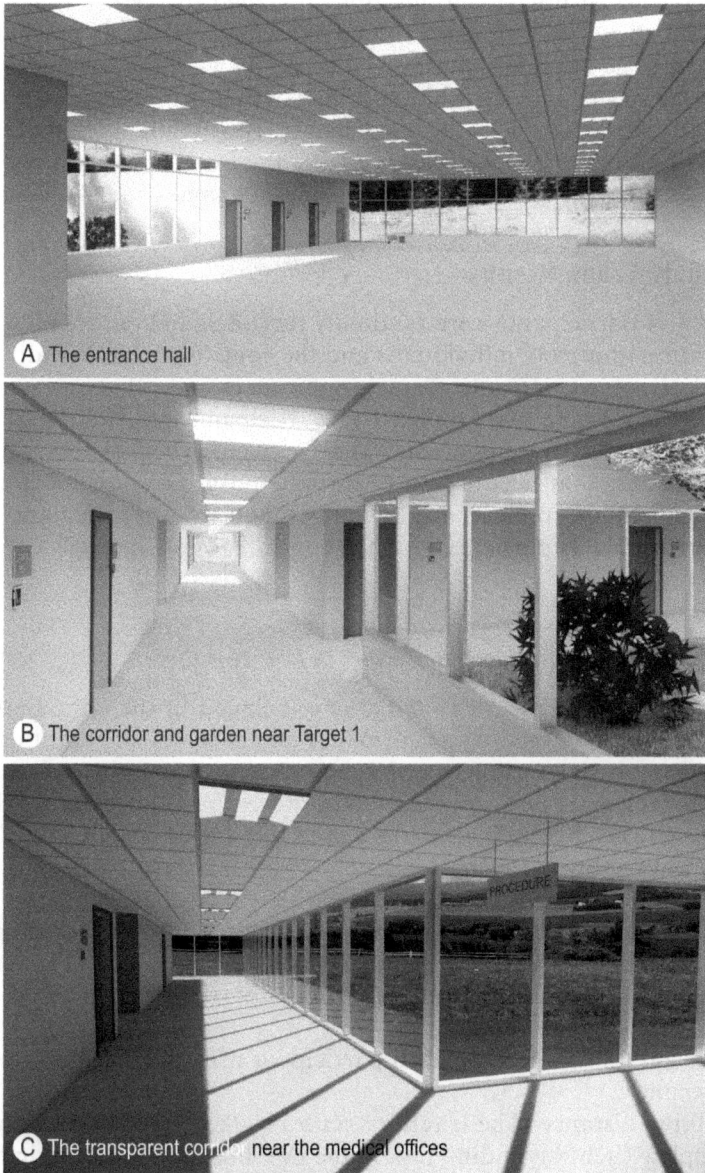

Figure 7.3 The real-time rendering and VR experience delivered to the nature group participants during the IVE wayfinding tasks, using the (A) the entrance hall, (B) the corridor and garden near Target 1, and (C) the transparent corridor near the medical offices, for example

Source: Drawn by Shan Jiang

environment (Schubert et al., 2001). Next, each participant was interviewed following a list of predefined questions intended to further explore one's wayfinding strategies and navigational experience in the IVE Wayfinding Task phase. The interview questions focused on what the wayfinding strategy was for each task and what specific environmental cues participants used to aid navigation. Finally, participants reported their computer usage habits and previous VR experience during the final Exit Questions phase, including the frequency of playing 3D computer games and VR exposure.

Data Analysis and Results

A total of 74 participants were randomly recruited and randomly assigned to the nature group (39 individuals) and the control group (35 individuals). An analysis of participants' demographic data indicated no significant differences across the two groups. Two participants quit the IVE wayfinding tasks earlier than the time limit due to severe cybersickness, a form of motion sickness that occurs as a result of exposure to immersive virtual/ augmented reality applications, which resulted in 38 participants in the nature group and 34 participants in the control groups who fully completed the experiment.

Wayfinding Performance and Behaviors in IVE Hospitals

Sixty-eight participants' video data were included in the data analysis to understand their wayfinding performance and behaviors; in addition to the two participants who experienced cybersickness, four other participants' data were excluded due to missing data or technique issues during the IVE wayfinding tasks. Six indicators were used to compare participants' differences in wayfinding performance:

*   Task completion: The number of IVE wayfinding tasks completed by each participant within the 15-minute time limit. This number could also be converted into the count of participants able to complete each task.
*   Task duration: The time each participant used in each task, reported in seconds.
*   Walking distance: The length of routes walked by each participant to complete each wayfinding task in the IVE hospital, reported in feet.
*   Stops: During the wayfinding tasks, some participants frequently stopped and looked around to reorient themselves when they felt confused or lost in the IVE hospital. These obvious stops during each participant's wayfinding process were counted.
*   Sign-viewing: When a participant's line of sight was intentionally pointed to any door sign (as indicated by the laser pointer integrated in the remote controller) during the wayfinding tasks (counts).

Sign-viewings can happen in association with stops or in the continuous movement condition.

- Ratio above optimal route (RAO): The ratio of the participant's actual walking distance to the length of the optimal route for each IVE way-finding task. RAO measures the efficiency of people's route selection based on the optimal route for any given task; a higher RAO score is presumed to be associated with a less efficient route selection.

Table 7.1 summarizes the statistical analysis of the identified indicators and compares the differences between the two experimental groups ($N = 68$) regarding participants' wayfinding performance and behaviors. A detailed data report can be found in Jiang (in progress).

A series of Mann-Whitney U tests revealed that participants in the nature group stopped and viewed door signs significantly less frequently than those in the control group during all IVE wayfinding tasks. Significant differences existed between the two groups of participants for wayfinding Task 3 in terms of task duration, walking distance, stops, sign-viewing, and RAO. Participants in the nature group used significantly shorter time ($U = 528.5$, $z = 2.01, p = .044, r = .27$) and walked a significantly shorter distance ($U = 557.5$, $z = 2.48, p = .013, r = .33$) to find Target 3 than those in the control group; they also stopped less frequently ($U = 624.5, z = 3.56, p < .001, r = .47$) and viewed

Table 7.1 Comparisons between the Nature Group (A; $N = 36$) and Control Group (B; $N = 32$) regarding Participants' Wayfinding Performance and Behaviors

Indicators	Group	All tasks	Task 1	Task 2	Task 3	Task 4	Task 5
			Individual IVE wayfinding tasks				
Task completion	A	27.00	36.00	35.00	31.00	28.00	27.00
(counts of participants)	B	19.00	32.00	30.00	26.00	20.00	19.00
Task duration (Md.)	A	447.50	52.50	70.00	82.00	100.0	33.00
	B	641.00	58.50	65.00	190.00	69.50	30.00
Walking distance (Md.)	A	1608.20	233.3	284.3	430.3	414.8	161.50
	B	2090.35	233.5	268.3	755.0	280.3	165.45
Stops (Md.)	A	24.50	2.00	4.00	4.00	6.00	.00
	B	39.50	3.00	5.00	12.00	6.00	.00
Sign-viewing (Md.)	A	30.50	2.00	4.00	7.00	11.50	.00
	B	52.50	4.00	8.50	15.00	8.00	.00
RAO (Md.)	A	1.67	1.05	1.37	2.22	2.27	1.02
	B	2.17	1.05	1.29	3.90	1.53	1.04

Notes: A series of normality tests were conducted on dependent variables, suggesting violation of the assumption of normal distribution. Considering the small sample size and severely skewed data distribution, Mann-Whitney U tests were conducted to compare the medians (Md.) of the independent variables (indicators). The grey cells represent statistical significance results between the two groups of participants on the designated variable using the traditional .05 significance level.

door signs ($U = 559.5$, $z = 2.51$, $p = .012$, $r = .33$) less frequently than those in the control group during wayfinding Task 3. Generally, participants in the nature group developed significantly more efficient route selection than those in the control group ($U = 557.5$, $z = 2.475$, $p = .013$, $r = .33$).

Task 3 was quite a representative task for testing the two types of hospital circulation spaces on general people's wayfinding performance. According to the results from the interview phase, for many participants, the floor maps played a fairly strong role in the initial two wayfinding tasks, and many participants could find the destinations relying on their memorization of the map. By Task 3, the impression from the floor map faded, and participants had a general understanding but not full comprehension of the hospital complex. Only those with very strong wayfinding capabilities could follow through Tasks 4 and 5, and the hospital was thoroughly explored by then, which also explained why there was a sharp decline in values for all indicators toward the final wayfinding task.

Participants' Mood States Scores

The POMS-Brief questionnaire was administered to each participant immediately after the wayfinding task. Three participants' data were excluded from the mood data analysis; two participants terminated the wayfinding task earlier than the time limit due to server discomfort caused by the usage of HMD, and one was missing data during the survey. A total of 71 participants' POMS scores were included in the data analysis. Internal consistency reliability evaluates the degree to which different test items proposed to measure the same construct produce similar scores (Streiner, 2003). The POMS-Brief questionnaire was examined regarding the internal consistency reliability as indicated by the Cronbach's alpha coefficient. The Cronbach's alpha coefficient for each subdomain of POMS-Brief fulfilled the requirements for internal consistency reliability, with tension ($\alpha = .898$), depression ($\alpha = .832$), anger ($\alpha = .873$), vigor ($\alpha = .860$), fatigue ($\alpha = .910$), and confusion ($\alpha = .740$) (George & Mallery, 2003). Table 7.2 compared the POMS-Brief scores on each subdomain between the two groups of participants. The results revealed that participants in the nature group experienced better mood states associated with the IVE wayfinding tasks than participants in the control group, including tension, anger, fatigue, and confusion. Nature group participants also experienced less total mood disturbance (TMD), representing more calming mood states, than participants in the control group.

Spearman's rho correlation coefficient was used to assess the relationship between participants' mood status and their wayfinding performance ($N = 68$). Table 7.3 reveals the statistically significant relationships between each subdomain of the POMS-Brief scores, task completion, task duration, and RAO for all participants. Medium-strength negative correlations existed between participants' tension, depression, and fatigue scores and the wayfinding task completion while strong negative correlations occurred

Table 7.2 Comparisons between the Nature Group (A) and Control Group (B) regarding Participants' Mood States

				Subdomains					
Mood states	*Group*	*N*	*TMD*	*Tension*	*Depression*	*Anger*	*Vigor*	*Fatigue*	*Confusion*
POMS-Brief	A	38	1.50	1.0	.00	.00	5.00	1.00	3.50
subdomain score	B	33	10.00	4.0	.00	1.00	4.00	3.00	6.00
Sig.	–	–		.030[a]	.071[b]	.324	.018[a]	.256	.082[b]	.004[a]

Notes: A series of normality tests were conducted on dependent variables, suggesting violation of the assumption of normal distribution. Considering the small sample size and severely skewed data distribution, Mann-Whitney *U* tests were conducted to compare the medians of the mood state scores.
[a] Represented a significant difference between the two groups of participants using the traditional (.05) significance level.
[b] Represented a marginal difference between the two groups of participants using a generous (.1) significance level.

between participants' anger and confusion scores and the wayfinding task completion. The results indicated that higher levels of negative moods were associated with fewer numbers of wayfinding tasks completed by participants. Medium-strength positive correlations existed between participants' tension, depression, and fatigue scores and the wayfinding task duration while strong positive correlations existed between participants' anger and confusion scores and the wayfinding task duration. The results indicated that higher levels of negative moods were associated with longer time spent in wayfinding tasks. A medium-strength negative correlation existed between participants' vigor score and duration. A small-strength positive

Table 7.3 Spearman's Rho Correlations between Measures of Mood Status and Wayfinding Performance (*N* = 68)

Scale		Task completion	Task duration	RAO
Tension	Spearman's rho	−.440**	.474**	.211
	Sig. (2-tailed)	<.001	<.001	.084
Depression	Spearman's rho	−.346**	.425**	.283*
	Sig. (2-tailed)	.004	<.001	.020
Anger	Spearman's rho	−.532**	.524**	.207
	Sig. (2-tailed)	<.001	<.001	.090
Vigor	Spearman's rho	.270*	−.355**	−.106
	Sig. (2-tailed)	.026	.003	.388
Fatigue	Spearman's rho	−.372**	.417**	.216
	Sig. (2-tailed)	.002	<.001	.077
Confusion	Spearman's rho	−.564**	.684**	.334**
	Sig. (2-tailed)	<.001	<.001	.005

*Correlation is significant at the 0.05 level (2-tailed).
**Correlation is significant at the 0.01 level (2-tailed).

correlation between the depression score and RAO and a medium-strength positive correlation between the confusion score and RAO were identified, with higher levels of depression and confusion moods being associated with less efficient route selection during wayfinding tasks.

Environmental Attractiveness and Atmosphere Metrics Scores

The 20-item EAAM questionnaire had excellent internal consistency, with a Cronbach's alpha coefficient of .92. An independent samples t-test was conducted to compare the average EAAM total scores between the two groups of participants. Preliminary analyses were conducted to ensure no violation of the assumption of normality. There was a significant difference in EAAM total scores between nature group ($N = 38$, $M = 63.82$, $SD = 14.08$) and control group participants ($N = 32$, $M = 53.78$, $SD = 11.41$), $t(68) = 3.23$, $p = .002$, two tailed. The results revealed that nature group participants rated the IVE hospital with transparent circulation spaces as being significantly more attractive than the control group in the windowless IVE hospital. Table 7.4 further reports the detailed response to each questionnaire item from the two groups of participants. Regarding the level of attractiveness, nature group participants found the hospital circulation spaces with sufficient nature views and daylight to be interesting, cheerful, pleasant, colorful, inviting, ornate, exciting, warm, and homey. In contrast, the control group participants tended to rate the windowless hospital corridors as boring, gloomy, ugly, dull, unpleasant, uninviting, plain, depressed, chilly, and institutional.

Participants also responded to two additional questions regarding their preferences for and opinions about the IVE hospital design. For the question "How much do you like the hospital environment you just navigated?", participants rated it on a 5-point Likert scale, ranging from 1 = "I don't like it at all" and 5 = "I like it very much." Independent samples t-tests revealed that participants rated significantly higher preference scores for the IVE hospital with transparent circulation spaces (nature group) ($N = 38$, $M = 3.54$, $SD = 1.108$) than the IVE hospital with windowless corridors (control group) ($N = 32$, $M = 2.25$, $SD = 1.008$), $t(68) = 3.223$, $p = .002$, significant at the .05 level. In response to the question about how attractive the IVE hospital environment seems (1 = "Not attractive at all," 5 = "Very attractive"), participants rated significantly higher attractiveness scores for the IVE hospital with transparent circulation spaces (nature group) ($N = 38$, $M = 3.54$, $SD = 1.029$) than the IVE hospital with windowless corridors (control group) ($N = 32$, $M = 2.25$, $SD = 1.047$), $t(68) = 5.18$, $p < .001$.

A one-way between-group multivariate analysis of variance (MANOVA) was performed to investigate group differences on three dependent variables: EAAM, TMD, and RAO as an indicator of participants' wayfinding performance. Missing data were excluded, resulting in a total of 66 participants' data being included in the analysis. A statistically significant difference existed between the nature group and control group participants on the combined dependent variables, $F(3, 63) = 3.72$, $p = .016$; Pillai's Trace = .15;

Table 7.4 Comparisons between the Nature Group (A; *N* = 38) and Control Group (B; *N* = 32) regarding Participants' Preference Scores to the Environmental Attractiveness and Atmosphere

Group and statistics	*EAAM itemized score*				
	1. Boring/ interesting	*2. Gloomy/ cheerful*	*3. Musty/ fresh*	*4. Ugly/ attractive*	*5. Dull/colorful*
A (*SD*)	3.05 (1.335)	3.03 (1.000)	3.50 (1.409)	3.29 (1.293)	2.50 (1.059)
B (*SD*)	2.41 (1.292)	2.22 (.975)	3.19 (1.491)	2.69 (.965)	1.72 (.958)
Sig.	.044*	.001**	.371	.033*	.002*
	6. Hectic/calming	*7. Unpleasant/ pleasant*	*8. Confined/ spacious*	*9. Frightening/ safe*	*10. Uncomfortable/ cozy*
A (*SD*)	3.68 (1.093)	3.68 (1.141)	3.63 (1.125)	3.89 (1.008)	3.24 (1.101)
B (*SD*)	3.22 (1.128)	2.69 (1.030)	3.22 (1.263)	3.59 (1.188)	2.75 (.916)
Sig.	.085[a]	.000**	.153	.255	.051[a]
	11. Drafty/still	*12. Uninviting/ inviting*	*13. Plain/ ornate*	*14. Tacky/ tasteful*	*15. Oppressive/airy*
A (*SD*)	3.61 (.916)	3.45 (1.179)	2.45 (1.108)	3.26 (1.223)	3.68 (1.068)
B (*SD*)	3.44 (1.105)	2.75 (.984)	1.38 (.751)	3.09 (.818)	3.38 (1.185)
Sig.	.490	.010*	.000**	.507	.255
	16. Depressed/ exciting	*17. Formal/ casual*	*18. Intimate/ distant*	*19. Chilly/ warm*	*20. Institutional/ homey*
A (*SD*)	2.97 (1.026)	2.84 (1.128)	3.29 (.956)	2.76 (.852)	2.00 (1.139)
B (*SD*)	2.28 (.851)	2.47 (1.016)	3.53 (.950)	2.31 (.931)	1.47 (.842)
Sig.	.003*	.153	.294	.038*	.033*

Notes: A series of normality tests were conducted on dependent variables with no serious violation of the assumption of normal distribution. Independent samples *t*-tests were conducted to compare the means of participants' mood states scores.
SD = standard deviation.
*Represented a significant difference between the two groups of participants using the traditional (.05) significance level.
** Represented a significant difference between the two groups of participants using the strictest (.01) significance level.
[a] Represented a marginal difference between the two groups of participants using a generous (.1) significance level.

partial eta squared = .15. When the results for the dependent variables were considered separately, the only difference to reach statistical significance, using a Bonferroni adjusted alpha level of .017, was the EAAM scores, $F(1, 65) = 11.37$, $p = .001$, partial eta squared = .149. An inspection of the mean EAAM scores indicated that nature group participants ($M = 64.67$, $SD = 2.15$) reported significantly higher levels of perceived esthetics and preference scores than control group participants ($M = 54$, $SD = 2.32$).

Level of Presence in IVE Hospitals

The 12-item IPQ questionnaire (Cronbach's alpha coefficient was .679) was administered to all participants at the end of the survey phase. Seventy participants' IPQ scores were included in the analysis; two were excluded due to early termination of the study, and two were missing data. Generally, all participants indicated a strong level of presence in the IVE hospitals, as indicated by their IPQ scores. The mean of all participants' IPQ scores was 7.5 based on a 10-point scale ($N = 70$, $M = 7.50$, $SD = .97$), and 68.6% of participants reported 7.0 or higher IPQ scores. There were no statistically significant differences between two groups of participants regarding their rated level of presence in the two IVE hospitals. There were no statistically significant correlations identified between IPQ scores and the variables that indicate participants' wayfinding performances or in their ratings of the environmental attractiveness and atmosphere of the IVE hospitals. However, Spearman's rho correlation analyses revealed that, for the control group participants, a medium-strength positive relationship existed between the IPQ and anger score, $p = .024$, $N = 31$, $r = .405$, and a medium-strength positive relationship existed between the IPQ and fatigue score, $p = .009$, $N = 31$, $r = .460$, both at the .05 significance level. The results indicated that higher levels of presence in the IVE were associated with higher anger and fatigue moods for participants in the windowless hospital corridors.

Preliminary Findings from Interviews

Each participant was interviewed regarding their wayfinding strategy in the IVE hospitals. The content analysis of the researcher's notes revealed five themes of wayfinding strategies and seven types of landmark usage during participants' wayfinding task. The five themes of wayfinding strategies included:

- *Strategy 1: Map Reading and Route Tracking.* Participants read and memorized the floor map as much as possible before entering the IVE hospital. During wayfinding tasks, they simply counted the number of turns, followed the left or right direction, then relied on the room numbers when getting close to the target. As one participant commented when trying to find Target 1: "I remember the second turn down the hallway and then turn left."
- *Strategy 2: Screening and Inference.* Participants developed a strong impression of the room numbers for each target. They first identified the corresponding range of the room number following the ascending or descending sequence of the numbering, then screened the room numbers to find the target. Participants understood the direction of unseen numbers based on inferences.
- *Strategy 3: Understanding the Spatial Arrangement.* Participants comprehended the overall spatial arrangement of the hospital after reading the floor map and briefly navigating the IVE space. They were able to find first the functional units where each target was located and then the target with the minor aid of room numbers. As one participant

commented, "I remember the overall layout was like, the radiology in the center, and all exam rooms along the edge."

- *Strategy 4: Relating Maps to the Built Environment.* Unlike theme 1, in which participants mechanically memorized the shifts and directions based on the floor map, theme 4 participants could always recall the floor map, associate it with the environmental information, and locate their real-time position in the IVE hospital. As one participant commented, "I have the map in my mind, and I just know where to go."
- *Strategy 5: Cognitive Mapping and Structured Paths.* Participants developed a clear cognitive map and structured paths in their mind for each task prior to the navigation. They were able to develop a pattern of routes and found the target efficiently. As one participant commented: "I followed an L-shape route for Target 1 and a horseshoe pattern near Target 2."

According to the existing literature, individual differences impact the strategies that people use in navigational tasks; however, nearly all individuals in certain circumstances have difficulty forming a large-scale cognitive map of a complex, unfamiliar environment, resorting instead to a less effective, narrow strip-like map (Baldwin, 2009; Rangel & Mont'Alvão, 2011). Therefore, strategies 1 and 2 are considered to be inherently less efficient than strategies 3, 4, or 5, which tend to formulate a more holistic cognitive map for wayfinding.

Based on the analysis of the notes taken by the researcher ($N = 69$), most participants relied on strategy 2 ($N = 30$) to find the targets, followed by strategy 3 ($N = 16$) and strategy 1 ($N = 11$), when navigating the IVE hospitals. Very few participants reported always being able to recall the floor map ($N = 7$) or develop a clear cognitive map with structured paths based on their understanding of the spatial layout ($N = 5$). The point-biserial correlation analysis was conducted to determine the relationships between participants' main wayfinding strategy and their wayfinding performance as indicated by the task duration and route selection efficiency (i.e., RAO). There was a statistically significant negative correlation between wayfinding strategy and task duration ($r_{pb} = -.454$, $N = 68$, $p < .001$, at the .01 significance level); there was also a statistically significant negative correlation between wayfinding strategy and RAO ($r_{pb} = -.301$, $N = 68$, $p = .014$, at the .05 significance level). The boxplots of task duration and RAO by wayfinding strategy indicated that participants utilizing strategies 4 or 5 tended to use a significantly shorter time and more efficient routes to complete the wayfinding task than participants using other wayfinding strategies (Figure 7.4).

Research evidence has supported that simply using signs in wayfinding is insufficient; the mixed use of salient landmarks, colors, architectural features, and environmental layouts warrants efficient wayfinding strategies. Beyond the use of door numbers to various extents, the content analysis of the researcher's notes also indicated seven types of salient landmarks that

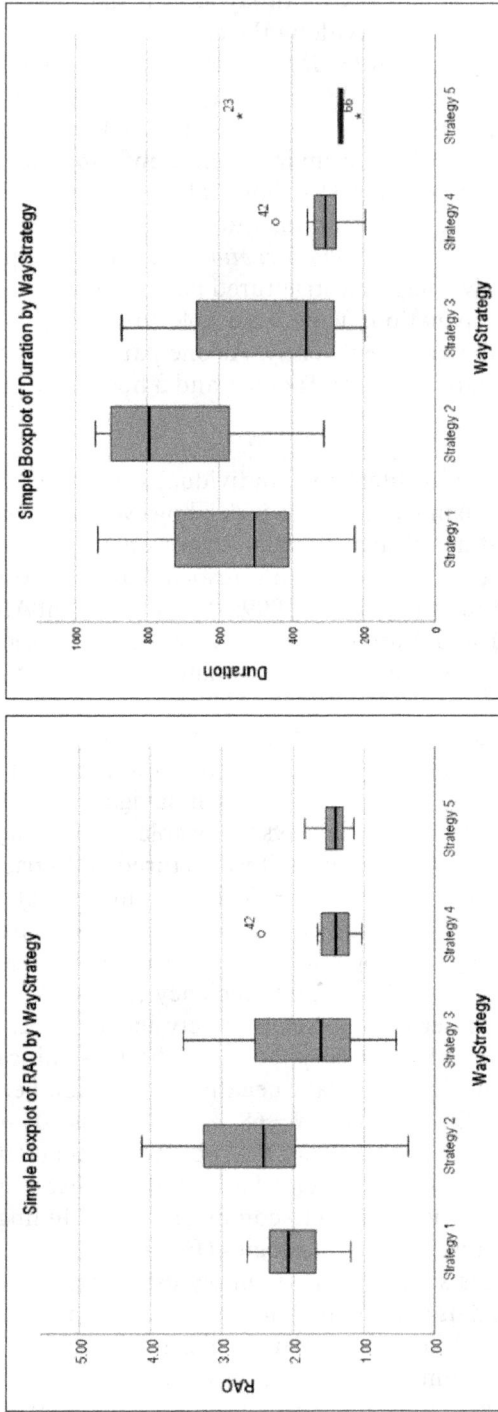

Figure 7.4 Comparison of participants' route-selection efficiency by the main wayfinding strategies (left) and comparison of participants' task durations by their main wayfinding strategy (right)

Source: Drawn by Shan Jiang

participants used to help navigate the IVE hospital. The seven situations of landmark usage strategies include:

- *Landmark 1:* Hospital gardens or window views to the outside nature
- *Landmark 2:* The radiology unit located in the center zone of the IVE hospital
- *Landmark 3:* The two main hallways along the east–west direction
- *Landmark 4:* Ceiling signs
- *Landmark 5:* Centralized nurse stations
- *Landmark 6:* The starting point near the entrance of the circulation space
- *Landmark 7:* None. No additional landmark used during navigation

Regarding the usage of salient landmarks, all participants in the nature group ($N = 34$) mentioned gardens or window views to the outside nature as one of the landmarks they used to aid navigation during the IVE wayfinding tasks. Other used landmarks in the ranking order include the radiology unit ($N = 15$), the main hallways ($N = 11$), celling signs ($N = 11$), the starting point ($N = 4$), and centralized nurse station ($N = 4$). In addition, 14 participants, all from the control group, reported that they did not use any salient landmarks beyond the room numbers during their wayfinding in the IVE hospital. A chi-square test for independence indicated a statistically significant association between garden/nature views as landmarks and participants' completed wayfinding tasks, χ^2 (8, $N = 68$) = 18.75, $p = .016$, significant at the .05 level. Participants who used gardens or views to the outside nature as landmarks were more likely to complete more wayfinding tasks than those who used other features as landmarks or no landmarks in the IVE hospital. The point-biserial correlation analysis was conducted to determine the relationships between participants' use of salient landmarks and their wayfinding performance. There was a statistically significant positive correlation between landmark and task duration ($r_{pb} = .266$, $N = 68$, $p = .028$, at the .05 significance level), indicating that participants who used garden or nature views as salient landmarks tended to complete all wayfinding tasks in a significantly shorter timeframe than participants who used other landmarks or no landmarks.

The interview results also indicated several obstacles that impacted people's wayfinding performance and experience, including the monochromatic interior design style as well as small door tags and room numbers that are hard to read from a distance. When asked about any spatial design features that could be added to help with wayfinding, nine themes emerged from the researcher's notes, which are summarized in the following bullet points in the ranking order, from the most to least frequently mentioned:

- Fifteen participants suggested including wall or ceiling signs with clear arrows to guide the way.
- Twelve participants suggested using unique colors to represent different function units and match the interior design style, decoration, and furniture to the color schemes.

- Four participants mentioned integrating ornaments, artwork, or murals in the circulation space to serve as landmarks during wayfinding.
- Providing lines and arrows on the ground to lead the way.
- Having a staff member in the IVE space that one can ask for help.
- Hierarchically numbering the rooms and integrating the functional units and floor information into the numbering system. For example, the 10th exam room in Exam A zone of level 1 in the hospital should be labeled as "Exam Room A-110," where A represents zone A, the left digit 1 identifies level 1, and the final two digits 10 represent the room information.
- Incorporating properly designed larger room signs to help people see the room information from a distance.
- Being able to see the floor map frequently, with the "current position" labeled, in the circulation space.
- Considering the spatial arrangement that has a central atrium space with the functional units arranged surrounding the atrium could help people orient in the hospital space.

Additional Takeaways

Before being discharged from the study, participants answered several exit questions, based on a 5-point Likert scale (1 = rarely; 5 = very often), regarding their previous VR and 3D computer game experiences. In terms of previous VR experiences, no statistically significant difference was identified between the nature group and control group. Similarly, no significant difference in previous experiences of 3D computer games was identified between the two study groups. The relationships between participants' (N = 68) previous VR/3D computer game experiences and wayfinding performances variables (i.e., task completion, task duration, and RAO) were investigated using Spearman's rho correlation coefficient. There was a small-strength positive correlation between participants' previous VR experience and task completion (p = .014, N = 68, r = .296) and a medium-strength negative correlation between participants' previous VR experience and task duration (p = .043, N = 68, r = −.246). The results indicated that more previous VR experience was associated with more completed wayfinding tasks and less time needed for the wayfinding tasks. However, the frequency of playing 3D computer games was not significantly correlated to the wayfinding performances in the IVE.

Summary of Findings from the Current Study

- Navigation and wayfinding in a hospital circulation space that has visual access to nature and daylight could significantly reduce people's negative moods, such as anger, confusion, tension, and fatigue, and help stabilize their total mood status, as compared to a hospital that has no natural views or daylight.

- Hospital circulation spaces with abundant natural views and daylight were rated higher preference scores by navigators in terms of the overall environmental atmosphere and the level of attractiveness as compared to windowless corridors.
- The integration of nature and gardens in a hospital complex could influence people's wayfinding decision and route selection as compared to the ones in the same hospital layout without visual access to nature or daylight. Gardens, natural views, and daylight attract people's visual attentions during their navigation in the VR hospital space. In hospital circulation spaces that have visual access to nature and daylight, people were more likely to choose the optimal routes or routes that were closer to the correct destinations. By contrast, in a hospital without natural views or daylight, people were more likely to select random and scattered routes, resulting in the opposite direction from the destinations during wayfinding.
- When experiencing challenging wayfinding tasks, such as finding a destination that requires three or more turns in a VR hospital (e.g., Task 3), people performed significantly better in a space that has visual access to nature than a space with no natural views. The better performances were measured as: less time consumed and shorter walking distance to find the correct destination as well as fewer stops and less frequency of viewing door signs during wayfinding.
- People were more likely to rely on the sequence of room numbers and door signs instead of other environmental cues to find their ways in a hospital without natural views or daylight. In contrast, people were more likely to have a better understanding of the overall spatial layout and develop a mind map with structured paths to aid wayfinding in a hospital complex that had abundant natural views and daylight in the circulation spaces. Gardens and nature views have strong potentials to serve as salient landmarks and improve wayfinding efficiency in the circulation spaces of a general hospital.
- Any inconsistent room numbering could be significant obstacles for wayfinding. People would prefer a hospital circulation space that has sufficient signs, maps, and arrows to guide their way. Color-coded interior design and matching furniture, art, and ornamental themes may aid wayfinding.
- People can experience fully immersive VR through a combination of advanced IVE techniques with the high levels of presence reported. For navigators in the windowless IVE hospital, when perceiving a higher level of presence and immersion, people tended to experience stronger negative moods, such as depression, anger, and fatigue, and more intensive mood disturbance associated with their wayfinding experience.
- Prolonged usage of the head-mounted display device through IVEs could cause slight to moderate levels of cybersickness, such as nausea

and dizziness. IVE techniques as efficient research tools may have strong potentials to manipulate people's emotional status. However, people's previous VR experience should be controlled when using IVE techniques in the future environment and behavior studies.

Additional Implications for Healthcare Circulation Spaces Design

Existing studies generally agree with four major spatial characteristics that influence people's wayfinding behaviors and experiences in complex building environments, including the complexity of the floorplan configuration (Haq & Zimring, 2003; O'Neill, 1991; Weisman, 1981); environmental identity or the degree of differentiation (Appleyard, 1969; Murakoshi & Kawai, 2000); environmental cues such as landmarks, signage, color, and affordances (Brown et al., 1997; Jansen-Osmann & Fuchs, 2006); and visual connectivity to the destination or other key locations of the environment (Arthur & Passini, 1992; Li & Klippel, 2016).

Beyond the scope of the wayfinding study documented in this chapter, research findings and design implications for healthcare circulation space design have been summarized from a series of empirical studies published in the recent two decades on topics of healthcare circulation spaces and wayfinding. Research findings are summarized according to the following themes, with the emphasis placed on the evidence-based design implications for circulation spaces and public zones in general healthcare environments; relevant findings from other types of facilities are selectively included to provide more insights for future design (Jiang & Verderber, 2017).

Spatial Configuration and Design Elements

- In healthcare design, systematic consideration of paths, nodes, landmarks, edges, and districts contribute to effective wayfinding and enhance users' overall experience. A clear hierarchy of circulation spaces (e.g., major thoroughfares, secondary stress, and back alleys) promotes exceptional wayfinding behavior. Urban planning and design principles are applicable to medical planning and hospital design, such as Lynch's (1960) five elements on the image of the city (Allison, 2007).
- People make optimum use of the expanded visual field to obtain navigational information; the optimized size and location of exterior windows or multilevel atrium spaces could expand the visual field beyond the typical limits in building interiors (Pati et al., 2015).
- Irregularly shaped and distanced corridors' intersections and physical obstructions are structural aspects negatively impacting the orientation and wayfinding experience. Rectangular unit shapes with linear pod alignments and perpendicularly connected corridors enhance movement and visibility (Zamani, 2019).

- Hospital staff members usually provide verbal directions that involve architectural features (e.g., hallways, lobby area) and environmental attributes and landmarks to aid patients/visitors' wayfinding (Pati et al., 2015).
- Certain characteristics of corridors in the birthing units can be frightening and cause anxiety, including (1) excessively long corridor arteries, (2) corridors with insufficient natural lighting, and (3) windowless corridors that lack visual connectivity with the world beyond. For corridor arteries, it is fear-reducing to provide connectivity with nature in a manner that allows patients, family, and visitors to circulate with relative ease into gardens and courtyards on site (Foureur et al., 2010).
- Integrating seating or nooks in a corridor for benches or ledges is preferred to accommodate the functional flexibilities and complicities (Carthey, 2008).
- The addition of a dedicated service corridor may help noise control, reduce staff stress, and improve staff satisfaction (Wang et al., 2013).
- The replacement of excessively hard surface flooring materials, such as carpets and high-performance acoustical ceiling, reduces "corridor activity noise" and enhances users' overall experience (Lau & Roy, 2014).

Environmental Identity, Signs, and Landmarks

- People in a large hospital environment frequently consult signs, maps, and landmarks or identifying anchor points for navigational information. People expect signs with high accuracy, the exact name of their destination on the maps, and a uniform pattern, height, and location of signs and maps across the hospital (Bubric et al., 2020; Pati et al., 2015).
- Signage is expected at eye level rather than near ceiling height; signage located above a door frame is less noticeable, and signs mounted closely to one another create clutter and information overload (Bubric et al., 2020; Zamani, 2019).
- The legibility of signs should be optimized through the appropriate font size to be legible from a distance as well as a strong color contrast between signs and the surrounding context (Bubric et al., 2020).
- An alphanumeric labeling system that incorporates building name/number, floor name/number, and room name/number in the system provides useful clues to hospital navigators (Pati et al., 2015).
- Color coding the routes to key destinations and visitor badges may help people address wayfinding challenges in the Emergency Department environment (Madson & Goodwin, 2021).

Wayfinding Systems and Technology

- People visiting hospitals who experience the frustration of an ineffective wayfinding system experience increased stress (Devlin, 2014). Interactive wayfinding displays in hospitals should follow the user-centered design principles, including classifying information according to user expectations, including a universal search, minimizing unnecessary onscreen information, adhering to platform standards, presenting visual aids effectively, orienting navigation information effectively, and providing environmental cues (Harper et al., 2017).

- Integrating technology is usually developed and tested outside the hospital and not as part of the overall wayfinding system design, which results in a mismatch in terminology, orientation, and effectiveness. Different wayfinding technologies face their own challenges; while mobile apps solve the kiosk challenge of avoiding cognitive overload, they result in a higher usage threshold. Any wayfinding technology should complement the environmental information such as color coding, landmarks, room and elevator labeling, and signage (Harper et al., 2019).

For Specialty Facilities and Vulnerable Patients

- Increasing complexity in floorplans has resulted in lower legibility of the spatial configuration, which has been found to negatively affect senior residents' wayfinding satisfaction in a care and attention facility. The circulation patterns should follow straight lines and avoid cross, grid, and ring patterns in senior care facilities Residents in an L-shaped floorplan that features one shift in direction showed less disorientation than those in H- or square-shaped dementia units (Marquardt, 2011; Tao et al., 2018).

- Environmental features that promote wayfinding among dementia patients can be implemented on two levels: the design of the floor plan typology and environmental cues including signage, furnishings, lighting, and colors. Building structures that support spatial orientation include small scale, direct visual access to relevant places, simple decision points and spatial anchor points, places with different and also legible function and meaning, signage, and personal items on residents' room doors. Information clutter should also be avoided to reduce confusion in dementia care facilities (Marquardt, 2011).

- Research findings support the value of variability in the architectural arrangement of circulation spaces and in "breaking up" long corridors. For dementia patients, architectural edge spaces and exterior walls with windows or views of nature serve settings for social interactions. Positive design interventions in hospital corridors include (1) removing obtrusive "institutional" features and instead introducing views of gardens and landscape features; (2) using opaque glass to accentuate the daylight while blocking out unsatisfactory external views; (3) changing the color/pattern of the ceiling, wall, and floor coverings to interject representations of nature; (4) reducing the width of corridors to a less institutional and a more welcoming scale; (5) introducing ergonomically designed timber beams to act as informal seating elements;

(6) planting trees outside, adjacent to the circulation artery and viewable from within; and (7) installing site-specific artworks at key intervals (Edgerton et al., 2010).

- The physical environment of common spaces and lighting use routines within assisted living facilities, corridors included, have an impact on patient socialization patterns. However, existing lighting conditions in many public circulation arteries of the assisted living facilities were assessed as inadequate; therefore, adequate lighting and abundant daylight should be thoughtfully designed in those spaces (Andersson et al., 2014).

- Suggestions for the improvement of corridor and associated circulation arteries in special care units (1) include the interjection of furnishings, color palettes, and works of art such as paintings to visually demarcate the end points of corridors; (2) include removal of extraneous equipment and furnishings from corridors to enhance fire safety preparedness, wayfinding, and spatial amenity; (3) incorporate furnishing at the end points of corridors, where feasible, to double function their use as nodes for social interaction; and (4) provide effective lighting yet in a manner that controls for excessive glare at the end points of corridor arteries (Topo et al., 2012).

- Environmental sensory cue recommendations for common spaces in assisted living facilities include (1) providing high contrast between surface finishing; (2) employing aesthetically attractive finishes; (3) using color, artwork, discernible graphics, and related memorabilia on walls to enhance wayfinding; (4) providing clear, well-placed signage; (5) providing effective visual/auditory alarm devices; and (6) avoiding distracting or confusing colors and graphic images on floor surfaces (Wood-Nartker et al., 2014).

- Visual impairments present obvious challenges in wayfinding. For visually impaired patients, specific signs near intersecting hallways could help navigation. The overall hospital lighting should be stably maintained at a high luminous level; the use of natural lighting through large windows should be controlled through blinds, and the floor materials/ patterns should be muted to reduce light reflectance or confusion. Creating perceptible pathways helps people maintain direction, such as a contrasting carpet leading to the reception desk (Rousek et al., 2009). Large open spaces in the hospital should be divided using partitioning and furniture to establish rectangular areas and clear pathways in the aid of wayfinding (Elbert et al., 2018).

Note

1. A peer-reviewed journal article related to this study can be found in the Health Environments Research & Design journal (Jiang, Allison, & Duchowski, 2021).

References

Allison, D. (2007). Hospital as city: Employing urban design strategies for effective wayfinding. *Health Facilities Management, 20*(6), 61–65.

Andersson, M., Ryd, N., & Malmqvist, I. (2014). Exploring the function and use of common spaces in assisted living for older persons. *Health Environments Research & Design, 7*, 98–119.

Appleyard, D. (1969). Why buildings are known: A predictive tool for architects and planners. *Environment and Behavior, 1*(2), 131–156.

Arthur, P., & Passini, R. (1992). *Wayfinding: People, signs, and architecture.* Focus Strategic Communications.

Baldwin, C. L. (2009). Individual differences in navigational strategy: Implications for display design. *Theoretical Issues in Ergonomics Science, 10*(5), 443–458.

Brown, B., Wright, H., & Brown, C. (1997). A post-occupancy evaluation of wayfinding in a pediatric hospital: Research findings and implications for instruction. *Journal of Architectural and Planning Research*, 35–51.

Bubric, K., Harvey, G., & Pitamber, T. (2020). A user-centered approach to evaluating wayfinding systems in healthcare. *Health Environments Research & Design Journal.* https://doi.org/10.1177/1937586720959074

Carpman, J. R., Grant, M. A., & Simmons, D. A. (1985). Hospital design and wayfinding: A video simulation study. *Environment and Behavior, 17*(3), 296–314.

Carthey, J. (2008). Reinterpreting the hospital corridor: "Wasted space" or essential for quality multidisciplinary clinical care? *Health Environments Research & Design, 2*, 17–29.

Cooper, R. (2010). *Wayfinding for health care: Best practices for today's facilities.* AHA Press/Health Forum.

Devlin, A. S. (2014). Wayfinding in healthcare facilities: Contributions from environmental psychology. *Behavioral Sciences, 4*(4), 423–436.

Dogu, U., & Erkip, F. (2000). Spatial factors affecting wayfinding and orientation: A case study in a shopping mall. *Environment and Behavior, 32*(6), 731–755.

Edgerton, E., Ritchie, L., & McKechnie, J. (2010). Objective and subjective evaluation of a redesigned corridor environment in a psychiatric hospital. *Issues in Mental Health Nursing, 31*, 306–314.

Elbert, K. K., Kroemer, H. B., & Hoffman, A. D. K. (2018). *Ergonomics: How to design for ease and efficiency.* Academic Press.

Foureur, M. J., Epi, G. D. C., Leap, N., Davis, D. L., Forbes, I. F., & Homer, C. S. (2010). Developing the birth unit design spatial evaluation tool (BUDSET) in Australia: A qualitative study. *Health Environments Research & Design, 3*, 43–57.

George, D., & Mallery, P. (2003). *SPSS for windows step by step: A simple guide and reference.* 11.0 update (4th ed.). Boston: Allyn & Bacon.

Haq, S., & Zimring, C. (2003). Just down the road a piece: The development of topological knowledge of building layouts. *Environment and Behavior, 35*(1), 132–160.

Harper, C., Avera, A., Crosser, A., Jefferies, S., & Duke, T. (2017, September). An exploration of interactive wayfinding displays in hospitals: Lessons learned for improving design. *Proceedings of the Human Factors and Ergonomics Society Annual Meeting, 61*(1), 1119–1123.

Harper, C., Jefferies, S., Crosser, A., Avera, A., Duke, T., & Klisans, D. V. (2019, September). Exploring hospital wayfinding systems: Touchscreen kiosks, apps and environmental cues. *Proceedings of the International Symposium on Human Factors and Ergonomics in Health Care, 8*(1), 172–175.

Jansen-Osmann, P., & Fuchs, P. (2006). Wayfinding behavior and spatial knowledge of adults and children in a virtual environment: The role of landmarks. *Experimental Psychology, 53*(3), 171–181.

Jiang, S., Allison, D., & Duchowski, A. T. (2021). *Hospital Greenspaces and the Impacts on Wayfinding and Spatial Experience: An Explorative Experiment Through Immersive Virtual Environment (IVE) Techniques.* Health Environments Research & Design. https://doi.org/10.1177/19375867211067539.

Jiang, S., & Verderber, S. (2017). On the planning and design of hospital circulation zones: A review of the evidence-based literature. *Health Environments Research & Design Journal, 10*(2), 124–146.

Lau, S. K., & Roy, K. P. (2014, July 13–17). Noise control in hospital corridor using evidence based design. *Paper presented at the 21st international congress on sound and vibration.* Beijing, China.

Li, R., & Klippel, A. (2016). Wayfinding behaviors in complex buildings: The impact of environmental legibility and familiarity. *Environment and Behavior, 48*(3), 482–510.

Lynch, K. (1960). *The image of the city.* The MIT Press.

Madson, M., & Goodwin, K. (2021). Color coding the "labyrinth": How staff perceived a two-part intervention to improve wayfinding in an adult emergency department. *Health Environments Research & Design Journal.* https://doi.org/10.1177/1937586721994593

Marquardt, G. (2011). Wayfinding for people with dementia: A review of the role of architectural design. *Health Environments Research & Design Journal, 4*(2), 75–90.

McNair, D. M., Lorr, J., & Droppleman, L. F. (2003). *POMS Brief form.* Multi-Health Systems Inc.

Medelita. (2017). Modern healthcare mega complexes are getting so large that people are actually getting lost inside hospital buildings. https://www.medelita.com/blog/lost-inside-hospital-mega-complexes-wayfinding/

Miller, C., & Lewis, D. (2000). Wayfinding in complex healthcare environments. *Information Design Journal, 9*(2–3), 129–160.

Mourshed, M., & Zhao, Y. (2012). Healthcare providers' perception of design factors related to physical environments in hospitals. *Journal of Environmental Psychology, 32*(4), 362–370.

Murakoshi, S., & Kawai, M. (2000). Use of knowledge and heuristics for wayfinding in an artificial environment. *Environment and Behavior, 32*(6), 756–774.

O'Neill, M. J. (1991). Effects of signage and floor plan configuration on wayfinding accuracy. *Environment and Behavior, 23*(5), 553–574.

Pangrazio, J. R. (March 1, 2013). Planning public spaces for health care facilities. *Health Facilities Management.* https://www.hfmmagazine.com/articles/418-all-access?dcrPath=%2Ftemplatedata%2FHF_Common%2FNewsArticle%2Fdata%2FHFM%2FMagazine%2F2013%2FMar%2F0313HFM_FEA_design

Pati, D., Harvey, T. E. Jr., Willis, D. A., & Pati, S. (2015). Identifying elements of the health care environment that contribute to wayfinding. *Health Environments Research & Design Journal, 8*(3), 44–67.

Rangel, M., & Mont'Alvão, C. (2011, September). Color and wayfinding: A research in a hospital environment. *Proceedings of the Human Factors and Ergonomics Society Annual Meeting, 55*(1), 575–578.

Rousek, J. B., Koneczny, S., & Hallbeck, M. S. (2009, October). Simulating visual impairment to detect hospital wayfinding difficulties. *Proceedings of the Human Factors and Ergonomics Society Annual Meeting, 53*(8), 531–535.

Schubert, T., Friedmann, F., & Regenbrecht, H. (2001). The experience of presence: Factor analytic insights. *Presence: Teleoperators & Virtual Environments, 10*(3), 266–281.

Seidel, A. D. (1982). *Wayfinding in public spaces: The Dallas/Fort worth airport.* Paper presented at *the 20th international congress of applied psychology.* Edinburgh, Scotland.

Streiner, D. L. (2003). Being inconsistent about consistency: When coefficient alpha does and doesn't matter. *Journal of Personality Assessment, 80*(3), 217–222.

Tao, Y., Gou, Z., Lau, S. S. Y., Lu, Y., & Fu, J. (2018). Legibility of floor plans and wayfinding satisfaction of residents in care and attention homes in Hong Kong. *Australasian Journal on Ageing, 37*(4), E139–E143.

Topo, P., Kotilainen, H., & Eloniemi-Sulkava, U. (2012). Affordances of the care environment for people with dementia—An assessment study. *Health Environments Research & Design, 5*, 118–138.

Ulrich, R. S., Zimring, C., Zhu, X., DuBose, J., Seo, H. B., Choi, Y. S., Quan, X., & Joseph, A. (2008). A review of the research literature on evidence-based health-care design. *Health Environments Research & Design Journal, 1*(3), 61–125.

Vogels, I. (2008). Atmosphere metrics: Development of a tool to quantify experienced atmosphere. In J. H. D. M. Westerink, M. Ouwerkerk, T. J. M. Overbeek, W. F. Pasveer, & B. D. Ruyter (Eds.), *Probing experience: From assessment of user emotions and behaviour to development of products* (pp. 25–41). Springer.

Wang, Z., Downs, B., Farell, A., Cook, K., Hourihan, P., & McCreery, S. (2013). Role of a service corridor in ICU noise control, staff stress, and staff satisfaction: Environmental research of an academic medical center. *Health Environments Research & Design, 6*, 80–94.

Weisman, J. (1981). Evaluating architectural legibility: Way-finding in the built environment. *Environment and Behavior, 13*(2), 189–204.

Wiener, J. M., Hölscher, C., Büchner, S., & Konieczny, L. (2012). Gaze behaviour during space perception and spatial decision making. *Psychological Research, 76*(6), 713–729.

Wood-Nartker, J., Guerin, D. A., & Beuschel, E. (2014). Environmental cues: Their influence within assisted living facilities. *Health Environments Research & Design, 7*, 120–143.

Zamani, Z. (2019). Effects of emergency department physical design elements on security, wayfinding, visibility, privacy, and efficiency and its implications on staff satisfaction and performance. *Health Environments Research & Design Journal, 12*(3), 72–88.

Zimring, C. (1990). *The costs of confusion: Non-monetary and monetary costs of the Emory University Hospital wayfinding system.* Georgia Institute of Technology.

8 Case Studies

This chapter demonstrates how the patterns presented and discussed in the previous chapters are being applied across a range of healthcare facility designs. Rather than introducing the entire project, the discussion emphasizes the inside-out relationships, transparent spaces, windows, and typical details in the reflection of literal and phenomenal transparency in the architectural and landscape spaces of a healthcare facility. Over 35 contemporary hospitals and relevant facility designs are discussed in line with the preliminary pattern language of transparent spaces in healthcare design, supplemented with brief explanations, images, or analytical diagrams[1].

Pattern 1: Hierarchy of Landscape Realms

According to existing empirical evidence, the higher greenery ratio in landscapes increases the likelihood of being a restorative medical campus favored by all occupants (Wang et al., 2019). The landscaped grounds set primers for a green campus and, therefore, should strategically incorporate a series of greenspaces through spatial transition and connection that are visible and accessible by all occupants. A hierarchical arrangement of the landscape realms provides solutions to a smooth spatial transition, unfolding the experiences of nature from a public central greenspace to a semi-public courtyard or atrium garden, a semi-private staff garden, and the private window view of nature from a patient's bedside.

Constructed on a previous soybean field, the Owensboro Health Regional Hospital (Owensboro, Kentucky) designed by HGA adopts a holistic design framework that integrates stormwater management, ecological reclamation, sustainable natural resource management, and human health through the hierarchical landscape realms on campus (Jiang & Kaljevic, 2017). According to the proximity to occupants, four hierarchies of greenspaces are clearly established. (1) Public realm: The restored grassland, interconnected retention ponds, and walking trail loops calibrate a green-blue palette for the public domain of the campus. (2) Semi-public realm: The Dry River Rain Garden offers a landscaped transition near the main entrance

DOI: 10.4324/9781003122180-8

and serves as a pleasant buffer between the parking lot and the hospital buildings. A commemorative garden featuring a distinct healing pond and a loop trail is located at the rear entrance of the building, adjacent to the cafeteria, offering nature experiences for staff members, visitors, and patients with mobilities. (3) Semi-private realm: The main courtyard garden is located in triangulation to the main entrance and the hospital gift shop surrounded by the medical building components. (4) Private realm: A rooftop garden in the women and children's hospital features an inspirational sculpture and luxuriant plant palette that promotes restoration. A small interior staff garden is dedicated for viewing yet offers an opportunity for staff members to rest and escape work-related stress. All levels of green spaces on campus collectively contribute to the therapeutic views and a fluctuation of nature experience for all occupants.

The Hierarchy of Landscape Realms pattern was also applied in the campus planning for Fiona Stanley Hospital in Murdoch, Australia (Hassell, 2014), in which a continuous landscape character is woven throughout the hospital precinct. A hierarchical landscape plan connects multiple levels of courtyards, piazzas, rooftops, parklands, and the extensive bushlands in an effort to reconnect people to the therapeutic nature and aid recovery. When lacking a spacious site for extensive greenspaces, the thoughtful configuration and orientation of the hospital building may borrow landscapes and views from a broader context (Cooper Marcus & Sachs, 2014). The landscape design for Provincial Hospital in Bloemendaal, Netherlands (2015–2016) included a contemporary application of a "ha-ha" (a classic element in the 18th century English landscape that uses a dry ditch to create a vertical barrier while giving the viewer of the garden the illusion of an unbroken view). The dry ditch in which a low wall is hidden separates the private terraces of the hospital from the surrounding park landscapes without breaking the visual continuity ("Bloemendaal Meer en Berg", n.d.).

Pattern 2: Courtyards that Breathe

Courtyards reconnect people to nature and daylight for those working in the functional units located deep inside the hospital block. Multiple courtyards in a dense building block break into the tedious envelope of the fortress-like building and make the interior spaces breathable. Breathable courtyards have become integral parts of REHAB Basel, Centre for Spinal Cord and Brain Injuries, Basel, Switzerland, designed by the architectural firm Herzog & De Meuron (1998–1999) in collaboration with August + Margrith Künzel (landscape architects). Two guiding principles underlie the architectural and landscape design for REHAB. First, different natural spaces are created that generate a variety of sensual experiences and aid spatial orientation in the building. Second, the landscaping should transcend boundaries and create connections between indoor and outdoor spaces as well as between different functional units (August + Margrith Künzel, 2003) (Figure 8.1). As stated by the architects:

> We have set ourselves the task of designing a multifunctional, diversified building, almost like a small town with streets, plazas, gardens, public facilities, and more secluded residential quarters.... The connection between indoor and outdoor spaces was our primary architectural concern.... From the main lobby, various inner courtyards provide orientation: one is filled with water, another is clad entirely in wood, the bathhouse is placed in the third, etc. You proceed along them until you reach your destination. (Herzog & De Meuron, n.d.)

The building integrates nine courtyards in its footprint to increase the perimeter wall, resulting in more than 65% of the building interiors being located in the daylight area within 15 feet of the perimeter wall. Ninety-five percent of all regularly occupied spaces have a direct connection to the therapeutic landscapes outside (Behringer, 2011).

The integration of courtyards and continuity of indoor–outdoor spaces can be found in many other healthcare designs by Herzog & De Meuron, including the Kinderspital Zürich (Children's Hospital in Switzerland) and the winning design proposal for The New North Zealand Hospital (NZH) in Hillerød, the largest hospital in Denmark. Herzog & De Meuron has invented a distinct language of hospital planning and design that sets them apart from the prevailing procedures with an emphasis on the arrangement of core functional units (e.g., operating rooms, pre-/post- operating supports, imaging, etc.) and the inclination of towers and vertical circulation. In contrast, hospitals designed by Herzog & De Meuron are horizontal, prioritizing the people–nature engagement and functioning like an introspective town. Taking the NZH design as an example, the campus incorporates a hierarchical arrangement of landscape spaces and courtyards into an organic, unconventional campus form that reflects biophilia and spatial fluidity. The plan for the 660-bedroom hospital is the integration of two seemly contradictory needs: the desire for gardens with views of nature from every room and the need for short internal connections. The continuous connection to nature accompanies the entire journey of visiting this hospital; paths in the fields lead the traffic to a hospital in the forest, and patients, staff, and visitors arrive at the center of the building in which the hall is transparent to the surrounding gardens. A total of 18 courtyards penetrate the building envelope, helping improve orientation and drawing views and daylight into the entire hospital (Frantzen, 2018).

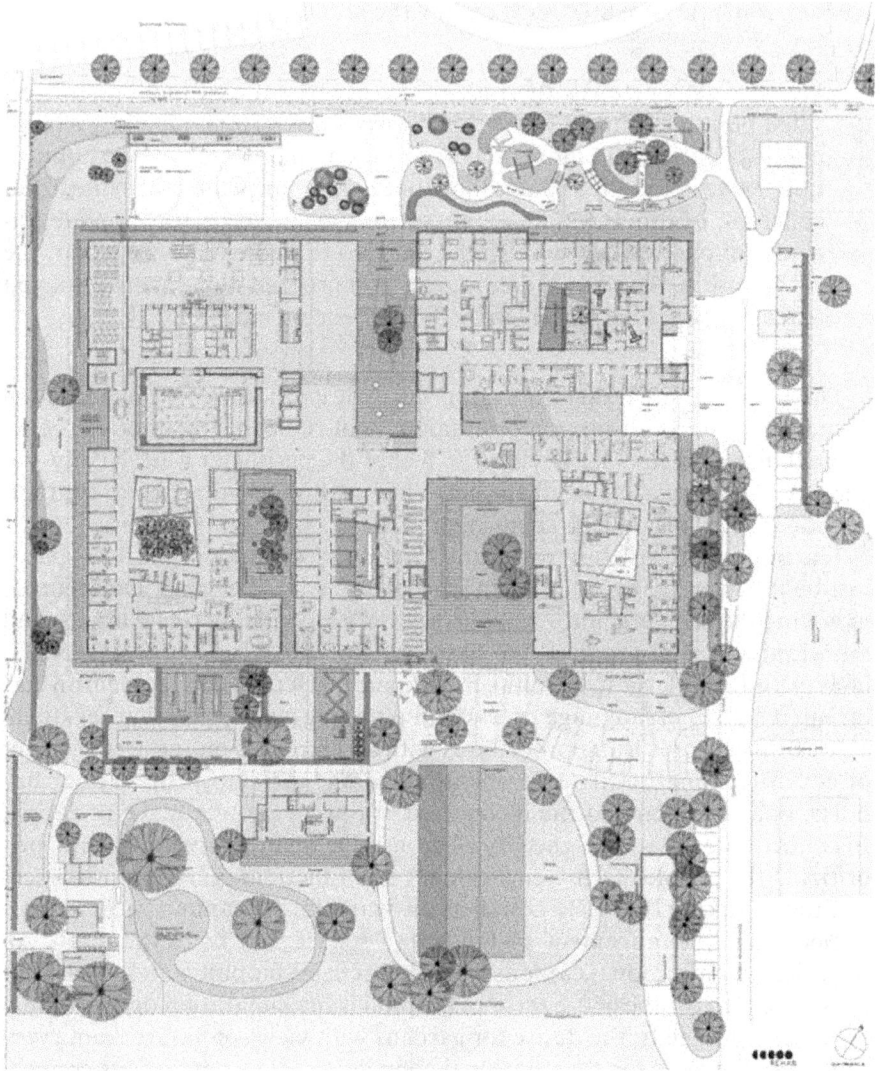

Figure 8.1 Site plan (left), entrance court with wheatfield (right A) and northern court with gledisia (right B) for the Neubau REHAB Basel in Switzerland, designed by Herzog & De Meuron (architects) and August + Margrith Künzel (landscape architects) *(Continued)*

Source: © Plan/Photo by August+Margrith Kuenzel Landschaftsarchitekten

A   Entrance Court with Wheatfield

B   Northern Court with Gleditsia

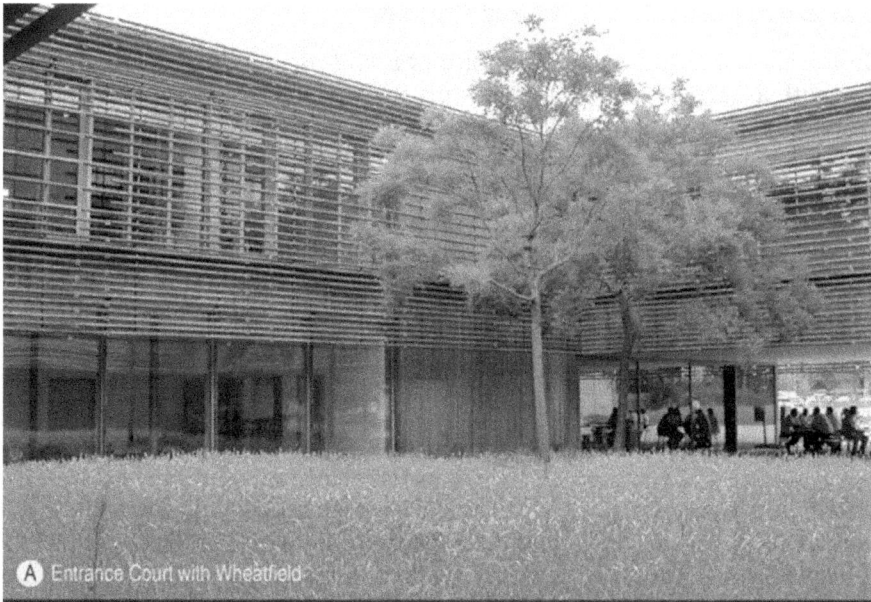

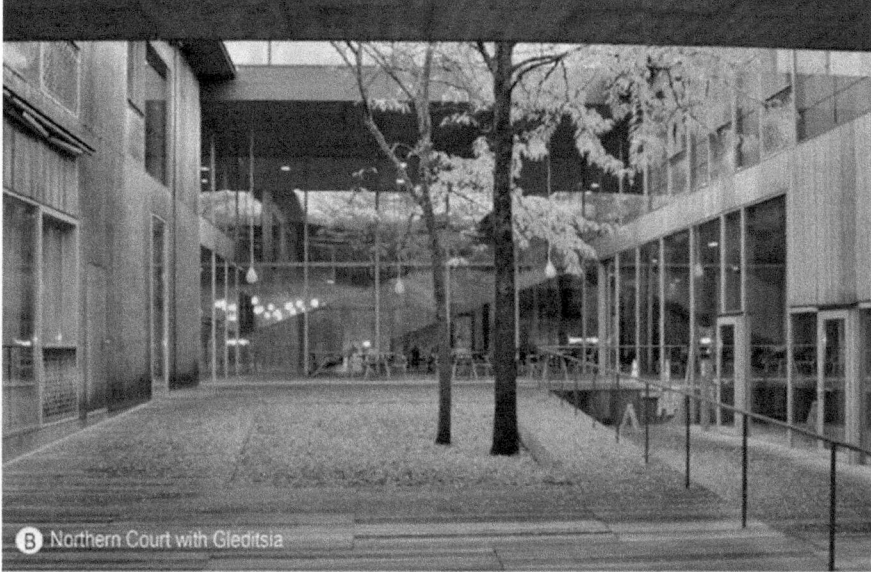

Figure 8.1 (Continued)

Pattern 3: Vertical Gardens and Cutouts

In the case of a dense site, the choice of a mid- or high-rise hospital building with a narrow footprint constrains the development of gardens on the
horizontal dimension. Vertical gardens and cutouts expand people–nature
contact beyond the ground level, introducing interesting views while offering "get away" opportunities for the occupants on the upper floors of the
tower. In the awarded competition proposal for a medical center for Firule
in Split, Croatia, the architectural firm Studio 3LHD (2009–2010) strategically planned acquired functions erectly, including vertical gardens and cutouts interspersed throughout all floors (Cliento, 2009). A façade envelope
in striated blinds pattern encloses the building, serving as the sophisticated
light regulator and sunshade while adding visual interests to the scenery
esthetics. The vertical gardens "divide and connect spaces of the polyclinic,
and instead of introvert hospital corridor, they provide a relaxing zone filled
with Mediterranean greenery, wooden terraces with views to the sea and
surrounding islands" (Studio 3LHD, 2009) (Figure 8.2).

In the proposal for the Gansu Provincial Women's and Children's
International Hospital Complex (Lanzhou, Gansu Province, China)
designed by SmithGroup, an on-structure, vertical garden system was creatively proposed to introduce nature views and accessible greenspaces to
the upper-level occupants of the patient bed tower. The six upright gardens
on multiple levels of the building form a vertical extension of the extensive
green roof terraces and segment the long building wing into two parts, providing visual relief and respite for patients and caregivers. At the TriHealth
Harold and Eugenia Thomas Comprehensive Care Center in Cincinnati,
Ohio, designed by GBBN, a generous central atrium features a three-story
living wall that demonstrates a healing landscape in the vertical dimension

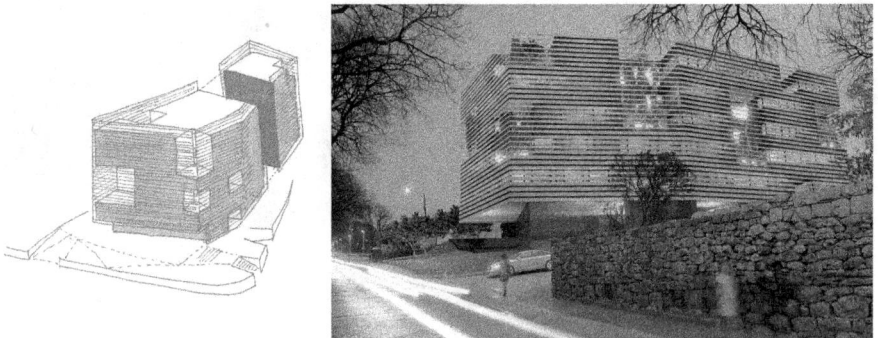

Figure 8.2 Rendering (right) and early-stage sketch (left) for Polyclinic St, a medical center with additional facilities in Split, Croatia, designed by Studio
3LHD (architect)

Source: © Plan/Image by Studio 3LHD

of the interior space. Six cutouts forming a series of vertical gardens are deliberately placed at the ends of major circulations, together with the windows at the ends of corridors, literally and figuratively lighting the way for patients moving between appointments (Morley, 2021). In the infusion clinic, views of the vertical garden, extending out to the treetops in the distance, keep patients engaged with nature during treatments (GBBN, n.d.) (Figure 8.3).

At the Dana-Farber Cancer Institute, Yawkey Center for Cancer Care (Boston, Massachusetts), a light-filled hospital building has been successfully established on a compact land in a dense city center. A 1,790-square-foot, two-story, glass-enclosed vertical garden—the Stoneman Healing Garden and Morse Conservatory—is visually and symbolically anchored around the building corner on the third floor. The garden is designed with plant structures, thoughtfully selected species, and a unique air-handling system following the strict infection control standard, providing year-round access to nature for patients, families, and staff. The conservatory overlooks the surrounding gardens on two sides, providing a protected sitting area for severely immune-compromised patients (ZGF, n.d.a). The garden provides therapeutic effects in aiding patients' cancer treatment and social and spiritual support along their healthcare journey (Dana-Farber Cancer Institute, 2012).

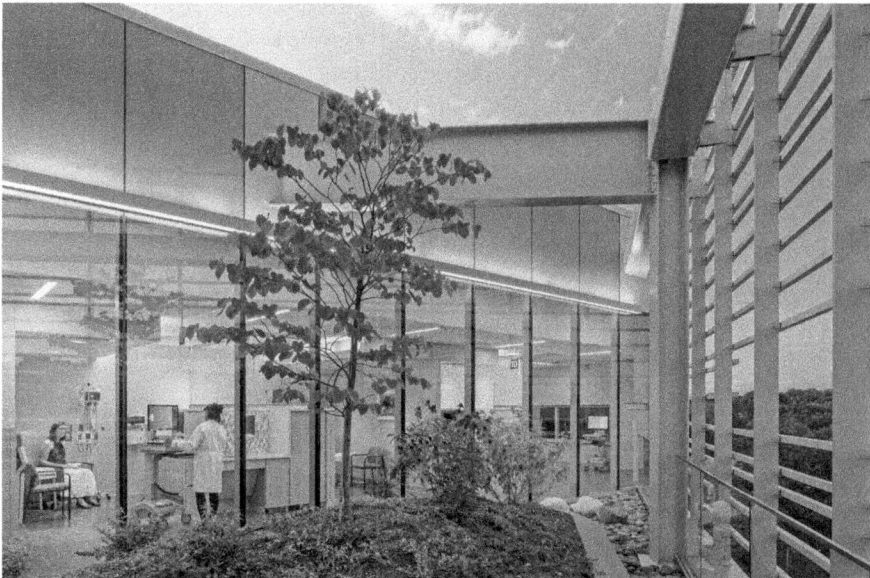

Figure 8.3 A cutout for the garden outside the infusion clinic at TriHealth Harold and Eugenia Thomas Comprehensive Care Center, designed by GBBN

Source: © Brad Feinknopf/OTTO (designed by GBBN)

Pattern 4: Positive Outdoor Spaces

As Alexander and colleagues (1977) discussed, an outdoor space is positive when it has a distinct and definite shape, which is as important as the shapes of the buildings surrounding it. Some degree of enclosure or convexity explains the positive characteristics of an outdoor space. Positive outdoor spaces are partly enclosed via structures or soft elements, and several paths leading through the space without weakening the sense of boundary. In the Kaiser Permanente Redwood City Hospital opened in 2014, the architectural firm HOK organized the buildings around a central open space. Two building blocks are intentionally staggered to introduce a positive space for a healing garden; the line of a disconnected landscape wall adds some degrees of enclosure along the edge of the garden, leaving one side of the space gapping to the rest of the open spaces on campus.

A central garden or smaller open spaces that lie between the buildings, in a positive convex and embracing gesture toward the buildings, usually lead to a positive quality of the space. In the Virtua Voorhees Hospital designed by HGA (Voorhees, New Jersey), the main hospital building adopts a curving form that embraces the landscaped campus and the preserved wetlands and pinewood field in the context of the site. A dining patio lies roughly in the center of the convex space defined by the building curve, between the main entrance and a staff entrance near the indoor dining court. The dining patio has become the most popular outdoor space and is consistently used by staff members, family members, and visitors (Jiang et al., 2018). In the case of Richard M. Schulze Family Foundation American Cancer Society, Hope Lodge completed in 2019, the U-shaped building encloses a positive outdoor space at the heart of the campus. The spatial layout is inspired by the cloister typology, focused on a central garden, to promote rejuvenation, healing, and wellness (Perkins & Will, n.d.a). A chapel is implanted in the outdoor space, immersing itself in the garden, which develops another concave–convex relationship nested within the positive outdoor space. A large yet lightweight roof in a grill pattern shelters the outdoor space, adding a layer of enclosure to the ceiling plane for the space (Figure 8.4).

ZGF architects have led the design of two medical campuses for the CHI Franciscan Health St. Anthony Hospital—one in Gig Harbor, Washington, and the other in Pendleton, Oregon—and both landscape designs were conducted by the landscape firm SiteWorkshop. The two campuses share similar design concepts and spatial layouts; building components embrace a central garden that promotes the overall positive quality of the campus's outdoor spaces, strengthens the inside–outside connection, and optimizes nature views. The Pendleton site had a challenging topography defined by a 150-foot grade change. The building is located at the top of the slope to take advantage of natural daylight. The hospital and medical office building are connected around a healing garden that features an upper-level ground with a composition of boulder outcroppings and native species; a stream flows

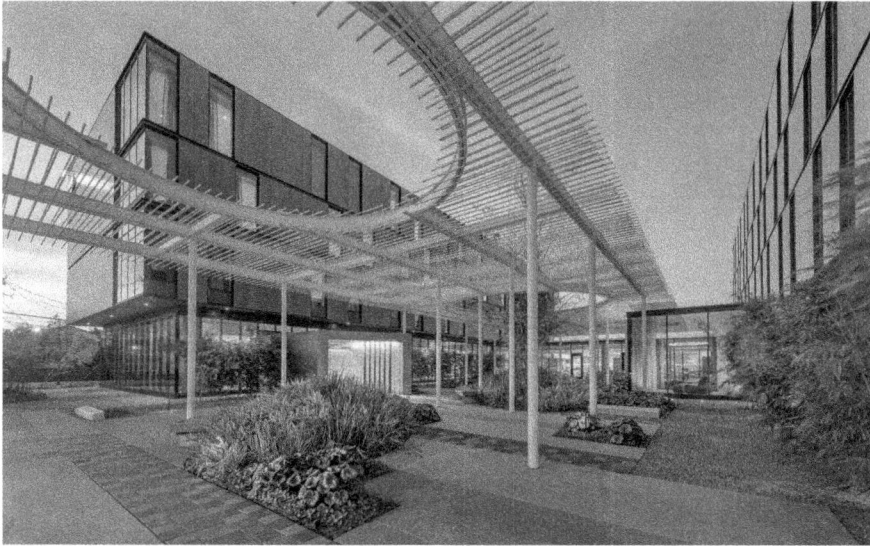

Figure 8.4 Richard M. Schulze Family Foundation American Cancer Society, Hope Lodge (Houston, Texas) designed by Perkins & Will

Source: © James Steinkamp Photography

down to a pond on the lower level of the garden, forming a lively yet soothing atmosphere for the campus (ZGF, n.d.b). Inspired by the Palouse landscape in the site context, the campus landscape at large involves extensive earthwork; rolling mounds of grassland were purposefully molded to block the unwanted views while adding interests for pedestrians when walking on the campus trails among the mounds. On the Gig Harbor campus, the building itself is nestled into the greenfield site, embracing a central healing garden visible from all main public spaces. The site design was inspired by the natural beauty of the wooded forest surrounding the hospital and "a walk in the woods" concept as a representation of a patient's journey from sickness back to health. Concepts such as exploration, silent reflection, moments of pause, and visual connectivity between interior and exterior landscapes emerged as design fundamentals and were further translated into design strategies that were applied to inside–outside relationships (ZGF, n.d.c) (Figure 8.5).

Pattern 5: Micro-Landscapes Along Narrow Wings

Narrow building footprints and shallow plan sections reduce the depth of the interior space and increase the degree of the interior space that can be daylit. Baker and Steemers (2013) discussed the importance of accounting

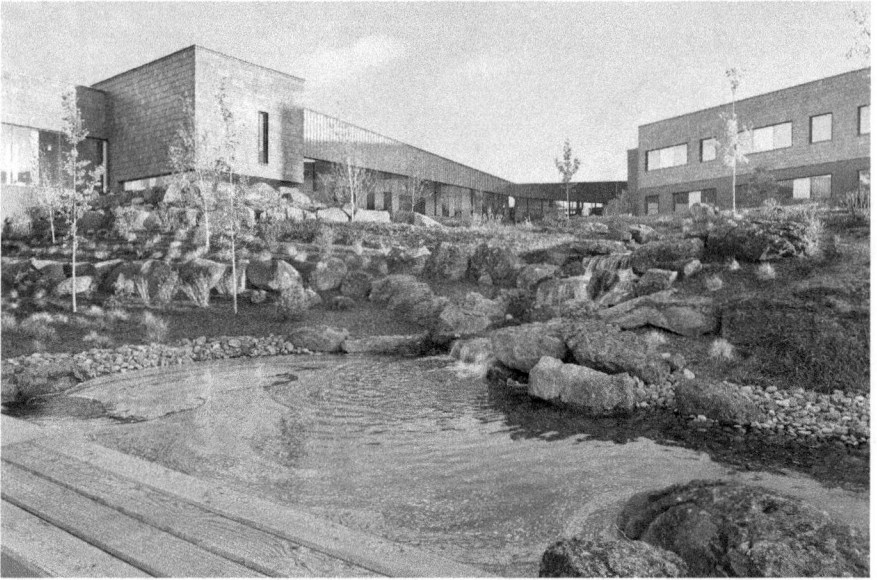

Figure 8.5 CHI Franciscan Health St. Anthony Hospital Central healing garden and water feature, designed by ZGF (architects) and SiteWorkshop (landscape architects)

Source: © Benjamin Benschneider (designed by ZGF Architects)

for a daylighting design as a primary consideration in the development of the overall building form. A rule of thumb for side-lit multi-story buildings is that a room can be adequately daylit for a depth (distance from the façade) equal to twice the floor-to-ceiling height (strictly twice the floor to the top of the window) (Baker & Steemers, 2013). Whenever the site condition allows, a building footprint that maximizes southern and northern exposures while minimizing eastern and western exposures should be adopted. A floor depth of no more than 60 feet from south to north has been shown to be viable for daylighting (Ander & US Department of Energy, 2016). Shallow plans in an overall large building can be achieved using courtyards, light-wells, and micro-landscapes to divide the otherwise thick plan. The pattern of micro-landscapes along narrow wings in healthcare design is widely accepted in European countries such as Germany, Denmark, and the Netherlands thanks to the building codes that require all rooms with occupants to receive sufficient daylight on a daily basis (Beermann et al., 2004).

A few design examples following this pattern include the Oslo University Hospital, Rikshospitalet (Oslo, Norway), Aabenraa Hospital (Aabenraa, Denmark) designed by White Arkitekter, and the original design and the latter extension of the Akershus University Hospital (Nordbyhagen, Norway) led by CF Møller Architects (2000–2014, 2014–2015). A common

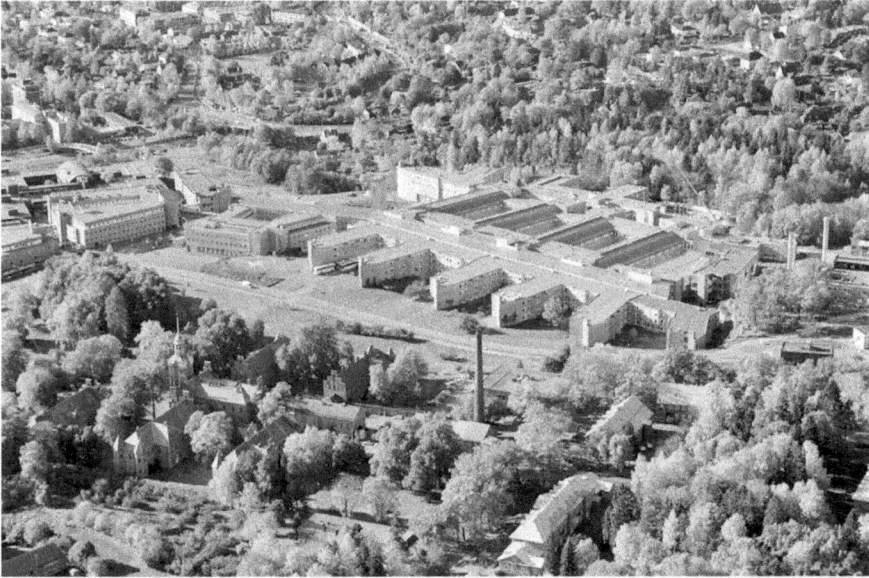

Figure 8.6 Narrow Wings at the Oslo University Hospital (Rikshospitalet) in Oslo, Norway

Source: © Lasse Tur

configuration shared by these hospitals is the linear, central spine that serves as the main circulation and public spaces; an array of narrow wings stretches out of the central spine, also described as the "comb structure" (Sunder, 2020), following a rhythm of arrangement and serving as the patient wards and different functional units. Micro-landscapes or courtyards separate the narrow wings, supplementing views and natural daylight to the hospital interiors (Figure 8.6).

Narrow building wings in geometrical forms and rectangular shapes can be speculated as the offspring of some of the older hospital plans, such as the courtyard hospital or the pavilion-style hospital advocated by Florence Nightingale. The narrow footprints and shallow plans can also be developed into curvy or organic forms. The New North Zealand Hospital (Hillerød, Denmark) designed by Herzog & De Meuron, as cited in Pattern 2, plans a 2-story ribbon of wards along the perimeter of the site and located on top of the examination and treatment pedestal. In the Gansu Provincial Women's and Children's Hospital project, two patient towers accounting for 2,300 beds are designed in narrow arc forms, positioning them on top of the extensive green roof terraces that belong to the medical podium on the lower level; all building wings follow the fluid curvy forms that surround the central green valley. Seven vernacular landscape typologies are represented through a series of greenspaces between the building wings—namely,

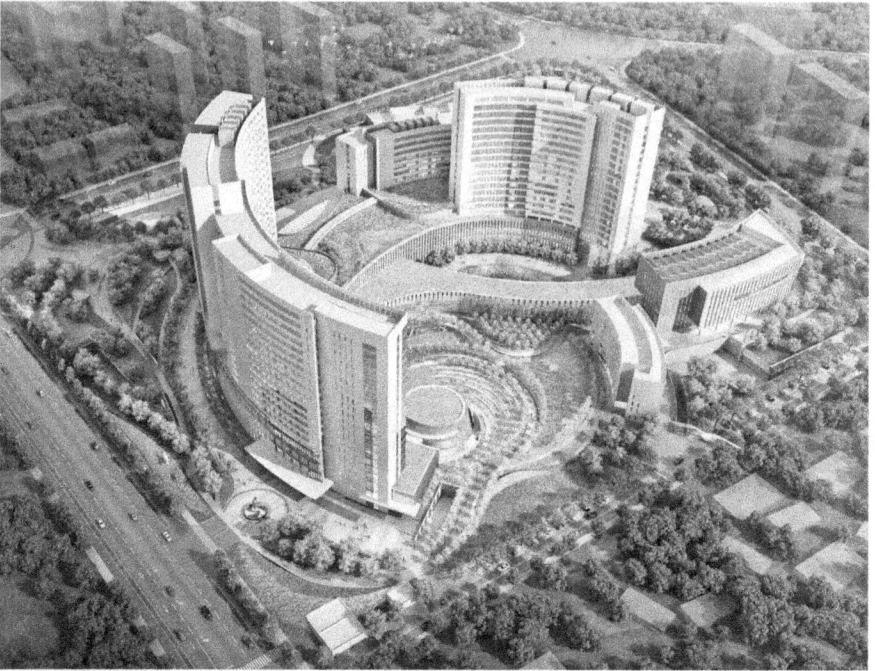

Figure 8.7 Gansu Provincial Women's and Children's International Medical Campus designed by SmithGroup

Source: © SmithGroup

"garden districts"—and connected by a pedestrian system on campus. The narrow building footprints substantially release areas for open spaces. The proposed campus plan resulted in 72% open space, more than doubling the city requirement of 35%, and the landscape areas account for 52% of the site (Figure 8.7).

Pattern 6: Cascading Roof Terraces

Compared to a single green roof, a system of greenspaces on top of several roof terraces could more efficiently improve the greenery ratio for mid- to high-rise buildings or a compact hospital site in the urbanized area. The Alder Hey Children's Hospital (Liverpool, the United Kingdom) designed by BDP (completion date 2015) creatively showcases an extensive green roof system for a large hospital complex. The design concept is a "hospital in a park": The building rises out of the green ground of the park on approach with an undulating profile, making it a striking iconic gateway to the city of Liverpool. A multi-layer green roof system product, Geogreen, finishes all of the roof areas, on both flat and steep curves and the lower-level roof terraces. The system incorporates a series of anchor points, a reinforcement geogrid, and geocellular technology to retain and stabilize the growing media and vegetation on the three curved roofs (ABG, n.d.).

Located on the eighth floor of the St. Louis Children's Hospital (St. Louis, Missouri), the Olson Family Garden, with a lead designer of EDAW is among the pioneering rooftop gardens and has thrived throughout two decades. The 7,500-square-foot roof garden features multiple layers of plants with seasonal interests, shading structures, various types of seating, and extensive water features, all of which could be challenging tasks for a green roof regarding the weight capacity, plant maintenance, and snow/rain day drainage. The permeable paving material allows water to drain through the drain mats and roof drains, which removes the water and weight immediately (Greenroofs.com, n.d.a). Right across the street, the latest expansion of the St. Louis Children's Hospital and the new medical tower for the Barnes Jewish Hospital incorporate four therapeutic landscapes for patients, families, and caregivers on accessible green roofs, echoing the Olson Family Garden. In designing each green roof, landscape firms Andropogon and DTLS carefully balanced "the rare and enlivening experience of the outdoors with medical and physical sensitives, such as allergens, light exposure, and skin and bone frailties" (Andropogon, n.d., para. 1). Each green roof was designed for a specific user group including a place for bone marrow transplant and other cancer patients; a garden as part of the maternity floor for new mothers and families; a children's garden for patients, families, and friends; and a private green roof exclusively for active labor and delivery (Andropogon, n.d.).

In the design of the Mary Catherine Bunting Center at Mercy Medical Center (Baltimore, Maryland), the new 18-story medical tower occupies a compact site, leaving limited spaces for green outdoors. Despite the oppressive volume of the overall building, a series of roof terraces defined by the building configuration ought to be credited to the project architect AECOM, and Mahan Rykiel conducted landscape designs in 2010 for the three rooftop gardens. Each rooftop garden has distinct design elements serving different user groups. The eighth-floor/maternity unity green roof features a lively water feature, commissioned sculpture, shady trellis, tables and seating, and a lush planting feature accessible by patients and visitors. The ninth-floor green roof serves the intensive care units, which provides a smaller garden with quiet, secluded seating areas. The tenth-floor green roof offers small planted area for visual access only. The roof gardens are visible from the medical tower and elevator lobbies, providing remarkable cues for wayfinding and spatial orientation (Mahan Rykiel, n.d.a).

The Khoo Teck Puat Hospital (KTPH) in Singapore designed by RMJM Architects in 2010 in collaboration with CPG Consultant achieved the optimal practice in the pattern of cascading terraces consisting of landscaped roofs, corridor planters, and planted balconies. Three medical buildings overlooking a central courtyard are integrated by eight roof gardens, five levels of corridor planters, and 81 balcony planter boxes. Each roof garden

portrays a unique theme curated by vernacular materials and plant species. Most rooftop terraces have been reformed to rooftop farms that cul-
tivate more than 130 fruit trees and vegetable plots, including more than
50 edible species (Greenroofs.com, n.d.b). Curtains of lush plants hang
down from the half-enclosed corridors and balconies as a waterfall of
greenery. The original concept of "the hospital in a garden" has thrived and
developed into a hospital in a forest: KTPH managed to achieve a green plot
ratio of 3.92, meaning that the total surface area of horizontal and vertical
greenery is almost four times the size of the land that the hospital sits on
(Kishnani, 2017).

Pattern 7: Transparent Arteries

Circulation arteries such as main corridors, hallways, and public transportation nodes should be designed transparent to the daylight and nature views
outside to increase the degree of people–nature engagement. An opaque,
enclosed artery could easily cut off the spatial flow between the outside and
the inside, leaving a disconnected experience of the entire hospital environment despite the existence of landscape spaces. Courtyards located near the
transparent arteries are more likely to be viewed and accessed by all groups
of users. In the Banner Estrella Medical Center (Phoenix, Arizona) designed
by NBBJ, a central spine includes a water feature and garden that separate
the patient tower and treatment areas, forming a canyon-like oasis between
the two structures. Corridors in double-story height enhance transparency
through horizontal stripes of skylights and windows, introducing natural
daylight to the upper levels and expanding the views to the outside on the
ground level (NBBJ, n.d.).

Patterns 5 and 7 compose a hospital building configuration that gives
priority to daylight and views, improves wayfinding, and is flexible in future
expansions. The Akershus University Hospital (Nordbyhagen, Norway)
adopts such a composition. A glass-covered main thoroughfare links the
various buildings and functions along two sides. The glass spine forms the
hospital's main arterial route and integrates indoor planting features. The
extensive wood materials in the interior design add a domestic feeling and
reduce the sense of rigidness typical of hospital environments. The transparent artery is also a major gathering space, structured as a series of open
spaces of differing character and a vibe of civic life, such as a kiosk, phar-
macy, hairdresser, church, and café (CF Møller Architects, n.d.).

In the case of the Lindesberg Health Centre (Lindesberg, Sweden), White
Arkitekter (2019) designed a timber building that advocates for a sustainable solution to healthcare architecture. The health center consists of two
buildings linked together by a double-story glass artery—namely, The
Gallery of the Senses. The glass gallery is transparent toward the sky and
allows for the spatial flow along the axis of the gallery and vertically. Living
walls and indoor plants add another layer of naturalness to the Nordic

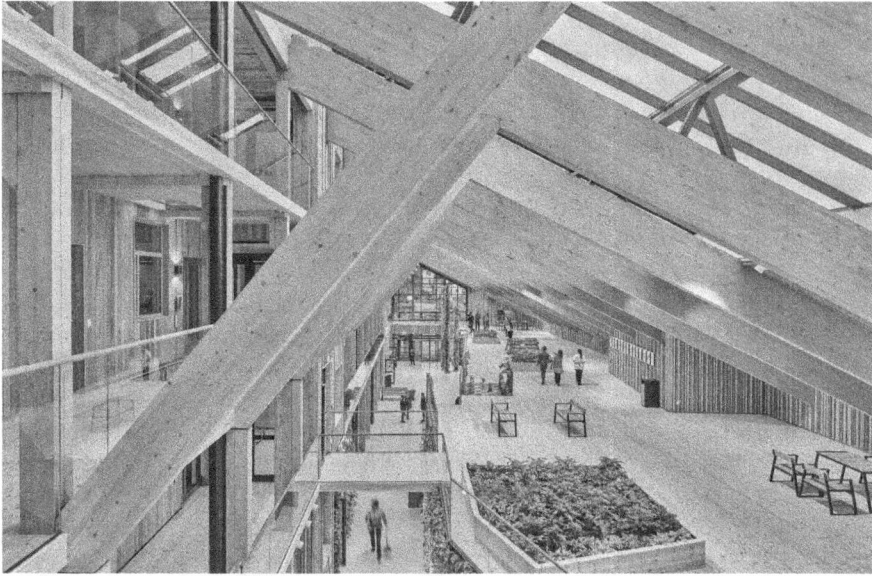

Figure 8.8 The Gallery of the Senses at the Lindesberg Health Centre in Sweden, designed by White Arkitekter

Source: © Åke E:son Lindman

timber characterizing the interiors (White Arkitekter, 2019). Similarly, a transparent artery has been implemented in the new research and education building at Alder Hey Children's Hospital (Liverpool, the United Kingdom) designed by Hopkins Architects (2018). Two modular wings house research and teaching activities shared by the NHS Trust and the university partners. The two building wings join at a curvilinear central atrium, establishing multiple connections between the institute and the surrounding park. The three-story design, central stair, and interior landscaping encourage internal circulation and communication through the building and minimize the use of the central lift (Hopkins Architects, 2018) (Figure 8.8).

Pattern 8: Landscaped Arrival Zones

Buildings with a graceful transition between the site and the inside are more tranquil than those that open directly off an unattractive parking lot. The experience of entering a building influences the way people feel inside the building. To avoid an overly abrupt transition, a landscape arrival zone is used as it is more likely to form a welcoming amenity and ease patients' stress upon arrival at the hospital. The entrance garden at the Kaiser Permanente Redwood City Hospital represents a landscaped arrival zone. In the Richard M. Schultze Family Foundation American Cancer Society,

Hope Lodge project, the entrance and reception open directly to the central courtyard and landscaping, offering a glimpse of the glass chapel that stretches into the courtyard.

The landscape firm OLIN (2012) designed the 6.25-acre landscape surrounding the Charlotte R. Bloomberg Children's Center and the Sheikh Zayed Tower on campus of the Johns Hopkins Hospital. An entrance court and gardens retained one-third of the football field-sized site for use as a series of gardens, "conceived as sensory-rich and visually simplistic spaces of orientation, respite, rejuvenation and calm for patients, visitors and employees alike" (Olin, 2012, para. 1). The landscaped entrance incorporates a water element, luxuriant planting features, and greenery islands that clarify the circulation pattern for patients, visitors, and staff, separating routes between the main entrance, children's entrance, and emergency drop-off. Rows of trees define the pathways, provide lines of sights, and soften the otherwise abrupt appearance of the main building complex (Figure 8.9).

In the University of Florida Health Shands Cancer Hospital designed by FLAD Architects and Sasaki Associates (landscape architect), two T-shaped buildings are symmetrically positioned, embracing a central park that consists of bioswales and a stormwater system. The buildings frame the main entry to the campus and provide strong spatial definition

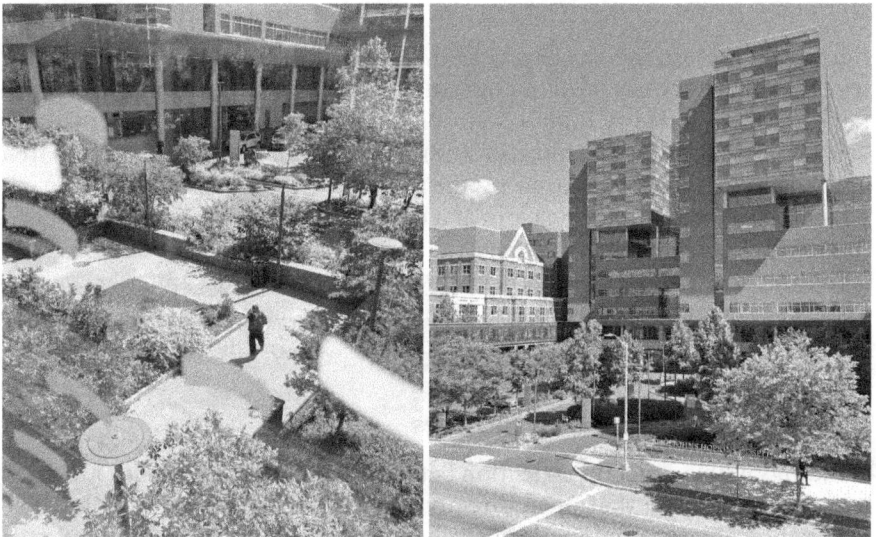

Figure 8.9 The entrance garden overlooked from the connecting bridge (left) and the landscaped entrance (right) at the new facilities for the Johns Hopkins Hospital (Baltimore, Maryland), designed by Perkins & Will (architects) and OLIN (landscape architects)

Source: Photographer: Shan Jiang

for the central healing garden (Rainey & Schrader, 2014). The main entry off Archer Road is marked with a four-lane entry drive planted with three parallel rows of palm trees, which have become a characteristic landmark aiding in wayfinding rather than needing to rely on signage alone. The passage through the palm rows also provides a presence of nature that is reinforced by the spray fountain and the view to the central garden. The palm drive ends at the central ponds and splits to either the main building entrance or the parking areas. If entering from the opposite direction of the site, moving along the contours of the ponds in the central garden easily leads visitors to the main building entrances. An entry orchestration is formulated: see, approach, arrive, park, enter (SAAPE) (Rainey & Schrader, 2014). The central garden and pond serve as salient features and visual anchors, reducing wayfinding difficulties in the beginning phase of one's healthcare journey.

Pattern 9: Dematerialized Edges

According to Verderber (2010), the exterior multidimensional edges of a hospital building can be highly porous, gridded, tactile, transparent, layered, and textured in contrast to the exteriors and edge conditions of the minimalist modern hospital that is often excessively institutional. In the case of Amami Hospital (Kagoshima, Japan), a 370-bed psychiatric hospital designed by Nikken Sekkei Ltd. in 2003. The aim of the project was to construct a "Lifestyles of Health and Sustainability" (LOHAS) hospital. The envelope of the hospital has been dematerialized, including the recessed windows behind a layer of porous screens that are composed of brick, concrete, and wooden ventilation grilles, known as the "wind terraces." Flat and deep eaves and the porous screens control solar radiation and ventilation for patient rooms, where patients can enjoy abundant nature, the changing seasons, and the flow of time on the site on Amami Island. Due to the dematerialized edges, natural ventilation, and daylighting design, the energy consumption of the Amami Hospital is approximately one-third that of a general hospital in Japan (Nikken Sekkei, 2008) (Figure 8.10).

In the case of Peter and Paula Fasseas Cancer Clinic, University of Arizona Cancer Center (Tucson, Arizona), CO Architect retained one of the existing abandoned facilities and adapted it for the new clinic. According to the investigation of patient and staff needs, consistent natural daylight was the most desired feature as the most common treatment of a cancer institute, infusion therapy, can take as long as 8 to 10 hours. The challenge was to bring natural light into the recesses of the original deep floor plan and offer vistas of the rugged landscape in the context of the site. The solution was to disassemble the building entity and cut three narrow courtyards/lightwells into the floor plate; the edges of all parameters of the building were dematerialized through deep eaves and recessed windows.

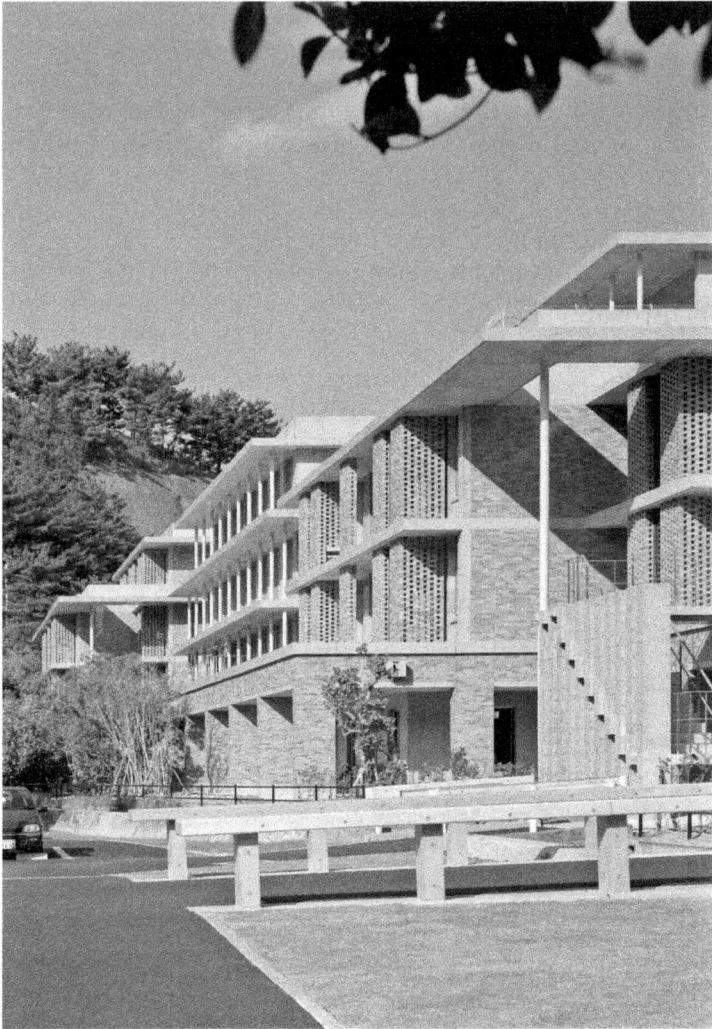

Figure 8.10 Amami Hospital in Kagoshima, Japan, designed by Nikken Sekkei Ltd.
Source: © Nikken Sekkei Ltd

Planted grounds extend from the courtyards to the window front; shade elements give light and shadow to the building but also extend the feeling of the building from the inside toward the outside, thereby integrating interior and exterior. An arroyo (dry creek bed) extends the length of the site, serving as a catch basin for collecting rainwater and condensate from the mechanical equipment, further augmenting the irrigation of the plants. The entire facility, including every exam room, infusion therapy room, and all

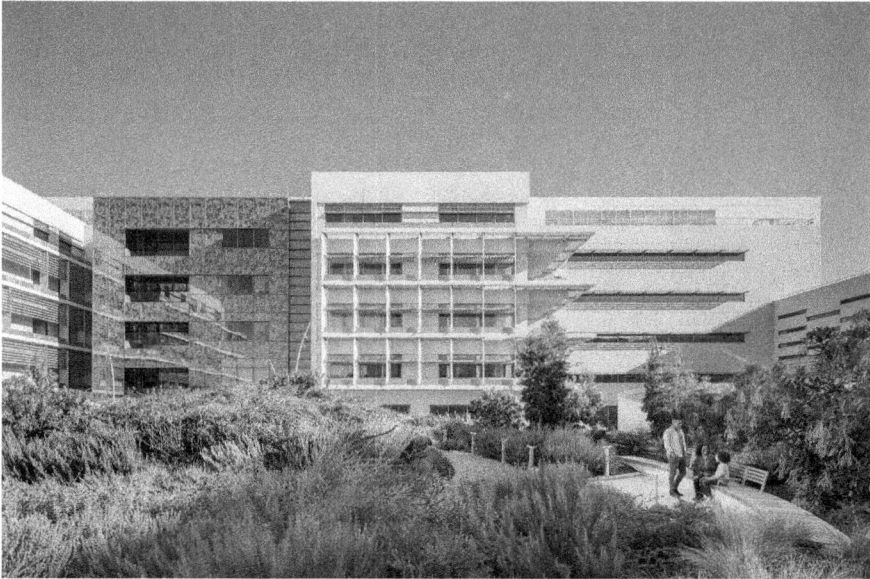

Figure 8.11 The Lucile Packard Children's Hospital Stanford's expanded pediatric
facility, leading designed by Perkins & Will

public spaces, is brightened as a result of the dematerialized building edges.
Scenes of distant southwestern mountains are visible from many windows
(HCD Guest Author, 2008).

The Lucile Packard Children's Hospital Stanford's expanded pediatric
facility, leading designed by Perkins & Will in collaboration with HGA
(executive architects) and Mazzetti (engineers) (2017), has achieved numerous merits regarding patient-centered and sustainable design (Figure 8.11).
The new hospital building has achieved LEED Platinum certification from
the US Green Building Council (USGBC) and is one of the five newly built
hospitals in the world to earn such distinction. The entire building was
designed with a dematerialized façade and edges; two outdoor terrace overlooks were integrated into each patient unit—one dedicated for patients and
family members and the other for staff members—allowing for convenient
access to fresh air and Californian mountain views. Window planters add
greenery and life to each child's healing environment while framing vistas
of the outside (Perkins & Will, n.d.b). The added overlooks and window
planters break up the often flat and rigorous façade of a hospital building
and diminish the institutional, forbidding atmosphere. Horizontal louvers
and vertical fins are installed on the building's façade at precisely measured angles corresponding to the sunlight angles, providing shade to the

interiors and reducing the need for air conditioning in patient rooms. The dematerialized edges and building façade, together with the innovative ventilation system in the design of the Lucile Packard Children's Hospital, has reduced energy consumption by 60% compared to average hospitals in the region (Perkins & Will, 2018).

Pattern 10: Atrium Gardens and Lightwells

Atrium gardens and lightwells effectively improve natural daylight and ventilation while diversifying the spatial experience in a deep hospital plan. An atrium garden serves as a harbor of refuge in extreme climates when outdoor activities are challenging due to excessive heat or cold. An entrance lobby/atrium symbolizes the start of a patient's journey in healthcare and deserves thoughtful design considerations. The entrance lobby at the Lucile Packard Children's Hospital (Palo Alto, California) features a 20-foot-high glass wall in an organic form with the interior design representing the scenery beauty and life of Californian shoreline. The transparent lobby overlooks the campus's central healing garden while filtering in ample natural light, contributing to a sense of calmness and serenity. The design was intended to invoke biophilia and place attachment, "making a child's understanding of nature an integral part of the healing environment" (Goodwin, quoted in Perkins & Will, 2018, para. 5).

The entrance lobby and central atrium at the TriHealth Harold and Eugenia Thomas Comprehensive Care Center (Cincinnati, Ohio), designed by GBBN, feature a three-story living wall that brings a vertical healing garden inside. The atrium, highly transparent to the outside landscape and the internal functional units, serves as the grand entrance and a central hub for gathering and circulation. From outside the building, the glazed atrium offers a stark contrast to the rest of the building envelope, like a glass heart seamlessly integrated into the body of the building. Inside the light-filled atrium, the continuous, wraparound walkway and stairs encourage physical activity and provide vantage points from which to survey the living wall and the entire atrium (GBBN, n.d.). A sculptural spiral staircase ascending two stories, together with the third-story bridge, offers people a mixture of sensorial experiences of light, shadow, and transparency as well as a variety of kinetic experiences in the public space. The central atrium/garden at the TriHealth Thomas Comprehensive Care Center has many merits that are comparable to the central atrium at the Cooper Union for the Advancement of Science and Art (New York City, New York) designed by Morphosis Architects in 2006. Both are highly visible and accessible public spaces connecting the institution to the physical and social fabric of the site context while fostering internal communications among different disciplines in the institute (Figure 8.12).

One or a series of smaller lightwells, not big enough even to allow people to walk inside, could efficiently draw in the much-needed daylight and views

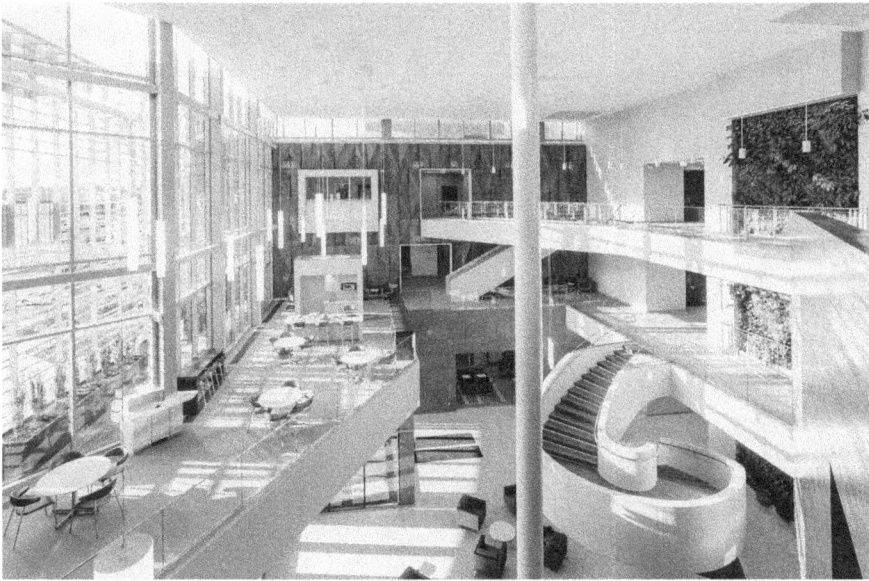

Figure 8.12 The entry atrium at the TriHealth Harold and Eugenia Thomas
Comprehensive Care Center (Cincinnati, Ohio) designed by GBBN

Source: © Michael Haas/GBBN

in a dark and condensed interior environment. In the case of Owensboro
Health Regional Hospital (Owensboro, Kentucky), a view-only lightwell is
attached to the staff lounge room, introducing daylight and nature views
while maintaining privacy and tranquility for the room. The women's
cancer center garden at Owensboro Health, a private, view-only rooftop
garden, serves as a lightwell overlooking the surrounding patient rooms.
The rooftop garden features rolling soil mounts, a lush planting palette,
and patterned grounds with beach pebbles and hardwood decking. A
female figure sculpture expresses hope and the uplifting spirit that encour-
ages female patients in recovery from cancer. In the first phase of design
and construction of John Muir Medical Center Walnut Creek Campus
(Walnut Creek, California), Ratcliff Architects gave special attention to
natural lighting design. The two-story lobby has abundant light streaming
in from the domelike clerestory windows. Patients and visitors on the third
through fifth floors have abundant daylight and views of a series of landscaped roof gardens. The interior public spaces are naturally lit wherever
possible; an exemplary lightwell features a pebbled island with water feature, rocks, and bamboo, manifesting a sense of serenity and meditation
as seen in a Japanese-style Zen gardens (Ratcliff, n.d.) (Figure 8.13).

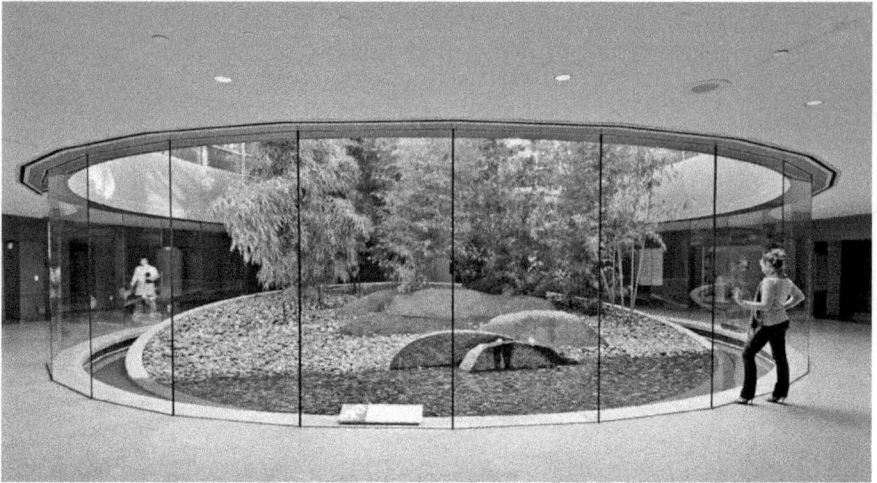

Figure 8.13 A lightwell at the John Muir Medical Center Walnut Creek Campus (Walnut Creek, California), designed by Ratcliff

Source: © Ratcliff, first published in Jiang & Verderber (2016)

Pattern 11: Sequestered Gardens

Unlike a central courtyard that conspicuously attracts people's attention, sequestered gardens are the greenspaces off the main stage yet thoughtfully planned that offer tranquility, soothing effects, or unexpected surprises for different occupants on a hospital campus. In the case of KTPH design, beyond the cascading green terraces and a central sunken courtyard, numerous sequestered gardens are important ingredients that contribute to the holistic forest-like environment. Navigating the hospital is comparable to an explorative journey in a jungle as one can hear the soothing sounds of running water from a distance but hardly see it until a sequestered garden in the first basement reveals a two-story waterfall "cascading into a deep pond, with turbulent and fast flowing water like that found in unpolluted rivers" (Khoo Teck Puat Hospital, 2016, p. 43). The pond and plants extend into the semi-interior space of the building, which is canopied by a deep eave, forming a continuum flow of nature-built spaces. Ornamental aquarium fish thrive in this waterfall pond; conditions in the waterfall feature, with dappled sunlight, good aeration, and many little nooks and corners, are like those in the jungle stream. The overflow from the waterfall pond is channeled into a stream that flows the length of the basement and ultimately enters the filtration system (Khoo Teck Puat Hospital, 2016) (Figure 8.14).

The sequestered gardens can utilize some pocket lots adjacent to the main building components. The Anne Arundel County Medical Center's

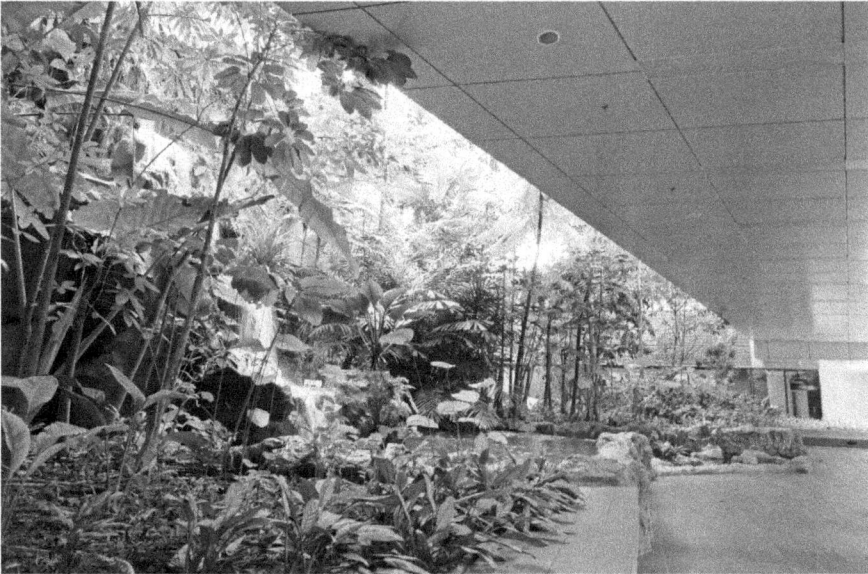

Figure 8.14 A sequestered garden in the basement at the Khoo Teck Puat Hospital in
Singapore, designed by RMJM in collaboration with CPG Consultant

Source: © Hancheng Wang

restorative garden is located adjacent to the Acute Care Pavilion, providing
a soothing environment for hospital visitors, patients, and staff. Although
the location of the restorative garden is near the building entrance, the entire
garden provides a sequestered and tranquil quality due to the enclosure
by the porous landscape walls along the garden parameter. The landscape
architects, Mahan Rykiel Associates Inc., filled the restorative garden with
luxuriant plants and shade trees as well as naturalist water features that rise
out of the rough textured boulders, transforming into a meandering stream
throughout the garden. Smaller parcels are defined by planting combinations
for multiple seating choices, which allows small group conversations in an
open area or individuals to find high levels of privacy (Mahan Rykiel, n.d.b).

Pattern 12: Therapeutic Viewing Places

The pattern of therapeutic viewing places should be applied wherever possible in a hospital environment. Implementing bay windows or large windows with low sills plus comfortable seating in the waiting, transition, or
other public areas contributes to the domestic quality of the space; views
to the outdoor landscapes at such places help relieve people's stress and
improve the sense of healing in the hospital environment. The waiting room
looking onto the Sr. Rita Peach Garden at Providence St. Vincent Medical

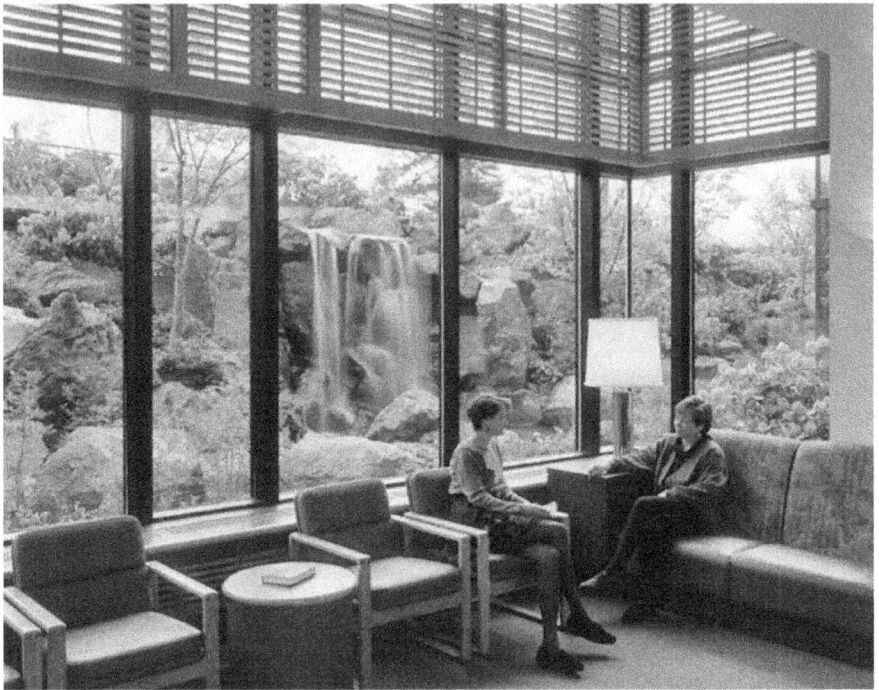

Figure 8.15 Providence St. Vincent Medical Center, Portland, Oregon

Source: © ZGF Architects

Center (Portland, Oregon) is a remarkable example of a therapeutic viewing place despite the rigidity of the overall configuration of the main medical building. At the St. Anthony Hospital in Gig Harbor, a generous public lobby with full-height curtain wall infiltrates overflowing daylight and the panoramic views of the central garden and the forest in the far distance. This pattern is combinable with patterns 2 through 11 discussed earlier in this chapter wherever a window is present. Several essential aspects warrant the therapeutic quality of the viewing places, including the level of transparency, the size of the window and the amount of views, the beauty of the view outside, and the arrangement and level of comfort of the seats. These aspects, together with other evidence-based design implications, will be thoroughly discussed in the following chapter (Figure 8.15).

Note

1. The preliminary pattern language of transparent spaces in healthcare design was first published in the article entitled *Landscape therapeutics and the design of salutogenic hospitals: Recent research* (Jiang & Verderber, 2016).

References

3LHD. (2009). Polyclinic St. https://www.3lhd.com/en/project/polyclinic-st

ABG. (n.d.). *Green Roof Case Study: Extensive Green Roof Alder Hey Children's Hospital, Liverpool, UK*. https://www.abg-geosynthetics.com/case-studies/green-roof-system-alder-hey-hospital-liverpool-uk.html

Alexander, C., Ishikawa, S., Silverstein, M., Jacobson, M., Fiksdahl-King, I., & Angel, S. (1977). *A pattern language: towns, buildings, construction*. Oxford University Press.

Ander, G. D., & U.S. Department of Energy. (2016). Daylighting. Whole Building Design Guide. https://www.wbdg.org/resources/daylighting

Andropogon. (n.d.). *How Can Our Landscapes Support the Patient Healing Process within the Urban Grid?* https://www.andropogon.com/project/washington-university-medical-center/

August + Margrith Künzel. (2003). *Neubau REHAB Basel*. Swiss-architects.com Profiles of Selected Architects. https://www.swiss-architects.com/en/august-and-margrith-kunzel-basel-binningen/project/neubau-rehab-basel

Baker, N., & Steemers, K. (2013). *Daylight design of buildings: A handbook for architects and engineers*. Taylor & Francis. https://ebookcentral.proquest.com/lib/wvu/reader.action?docID=1588412&ppg=54

Beermann, B., Henke, N., Brenscheidt, F., & Windel, A. (Eds.). (September, 2004). *Well-being in the office – Health and safety at work in the office*. Federal Institute for Occupational Safety and Health, in cooperation with the European Network—Workplace Health Promotion (ENWHP)

Behringer, E. (2011). *The daylight imperative* [Unpublished master's thesis]. Clemson University. https://tigerprints.clemson.edu/all_theses/1120

Bloemendaal Meer en Berg. (n.d.). *Hosper*. https://www.hosper.nl/tuinen-en-terreinen/bloemendaal-meer-en-berg/

CF Møller Architects. (n.d.). *Akershus University Hospital (New Ahus)*. https://www.cfmoller.com/p/Akershus-University-Hospital-New-Ahus-i269.html

Cliento, K. (2009, July 24). Polyclinic/3LHD Architects. *ArchDaily*. https://www.archdaily.com/30089/polyclinic-3ldh-architects

Cooper Marcus, C., & Sachs, N. A. (2014). *Therapeutic landscapes: An evidence-based approach to designing healing gardens and restorative outdoor spaces*. John Wiley & Sons.

Dana-Farber Cancer Institute. (2012, February 16). *How Our Patients Help Create a Healing Environment*. https://blog.dana-farber.org/insight/2012/02/how-our-patients-help-create-a-healing-environment/

Frantzen, J. (2018). *Herzog & de Meuron: New North Zealand Hospital* [Video]. Vimeo. https://vimeo.com/418366861

GBBN. (n.d.). *A Community of Care. TriHealth, Harold M. and Eugenia S. Thomas Comprehensive Care Center*. https://www.gbbn.com/work/trihealth-harold-m-and-eugenia-s-thomas-comprehensive-care-center/?backProjectType=63

Greenroofs.com. (n.d.a). *Olson Family Garden, St. Louis Children's Hospital*. https://www.greenroofs.com/projects/olson-family-garden-st-louis-childrens-hospital/

Greenroofs.com. (n.d.b). *Khoo Teck Puat Hospital (KTPH)*. https://living-future.org/biophilic/case-studies/award-winner-khoo-teck-puat-hospital/

Hassell. (2014). *Fiona Stanley Hospital*. https://www.hassellstudio.com/project/fiona-stanley-hospital#0

HCD Guest Author. (2008, October 31). Peter and Paula Fasseas Cancer Clinic at University Medical Center North Tucson, Arizona CO Architects. *Healthcare Design*. https://healthcaredesignmagazine.com/architecture/peter-and-paula-fasseas-cancer-clinic-university-medical-center-north-tucson-arizona-co-arch/

Herzog & De Meuron. (n.d.). *165 Rehab Basel, Centre for Spinal Cord and Brain Injuries.* https://www.herzogdemeuron.com/index/projects/complete-works/151-175/165-rehab-centre-for-spinal-cord-and-brain-injuries.html

Hopkins Architects. (2018). *Alder Hey Children's Hospital: Institute in the Park.* https://www.hopkins.co.uk/projects/4/205/

Jiang, S., & Kaljevic, S. (2017). Owensboro Health Regional Hospital. *Landscape performance series*. Landscape Architecture Foundation. https://doi.org/10.31353/cs1210

Jiang, S., Staloch, K., & Kaljevic, S. (2018). Opportunities and barriers to using hospital gardens: Comparative post occupancy evaluations of healthcare landscape environments. *Journal of Therapeutic Horticulture, 28*(2), 23–56.

Jiang, S., & Verderber, S. (2016). Landscape therapeutics and the design of salutogenic hospitals: Recent research. *World Health Design, 8*(2), 40–51.

Khoo Teck Puat Hospital. (2016). *A healing space: Creating biodiversity at Khoo Teck Puat Hospital*. Corporate Communications Department, Alexandra Health System. https://issuu.com/yishunhealth/docs/ktph_a_healing_space

Kishnani, N. (2017, September 8). Singapore's Khoo Teck Puat Hospital: Biophilic design in action. *Interface*. https://blog.interface.com/khoo-teck-puat-hospital-singapore-biophilic-design/

Mahan Rykiel. (n.d.a). *Mary Catherine Bunting Center at Mercy Medical Center.* https://www.mahanrykiel.com/portfolio/mercy-medical-center/

Mahan Rykiel. (n.d.b) *Anne Arundel Medical Center Restorative Garden.* https://www.mahanrykiel.com/portfolio/anne-arundel-medical-center-healing-garden/

Morley, J. B. (2021, March 5). Biophilia takes precedence at the TriHealth Harold and Eugenia Thomas Comprehensive Care Center. *The Architect's Newspaper.* https://www.archpaper.com/2021/03/biophilia-takes-precedence-trihealth-harold-and-eugenia-thomas-comprehensive-care-center/

NBBJ. (n.d.). *Banner Estrella Medical Center.* https://d3pxppq3195xue.cloudfront.net/media/files/Banner_Estrella_nbbj_case_study.pdf

Nikken Sekkei. (2008, September 21–25). *Amami Hospital, Kagoshima, Japan*. 2008 World Sustainable Building Conference (World SB08 Melbourne), Melbourne, Australia. https://www.ibec.or.jp/CASBEE/english/SB08_pdf/Nikken_Amami_Hospital.pdf

Olin. (2012). *The Johns Hopkins Hospital Entry Courtyard and Gardens*. https://www.theolinstudio.com/johns-hopkins-hospital-entry-court-and-phipps-garden

Perkins & Will. (n.d.a). *Richard M. Schulze Family Foundation American Cancer Society, Hope Lodge*. https://perkinswill.com/project/hope-lodge-houston/

Perkins & Will. (n.d.b). *Lucile Packard Children's Hospital Stanford.* https://perkinswill.com/project/lucile-packard-childrens-hospital-stanford/

Perkins & Will. (2018). *Lucile Packard Children's Hospital Stanford Achieves LEED Platinum Certification.* https://perkinswill.com/news/perkinswill-designed-childrens-hospital-achieves-leed-platinum-certification/

Rainey, R. M., & Schrader, A. K. (2014). *Architecture as medicine: The UF Health Shands Cancer Hospital, a case study*. University of Virginia Press.

Ratcliff. (n.d.). *John Muir Health Master Plan, Expansion and Remodel.* https://ratcliffarch.com/projects/john-muir-health-master-plan-expansion-and-remodel/

Sunder, W. (2020). *The patient room: Planning, design, layout.* Birkäuser.

Verderber, S. (2010). *Innovations in hospital architecture.* Routledge.

Wang, R., Zhao, J., Meitner, M. J., Hu, Y., & Xu, X. (2019). Characteristics of urban green spaces in relation to aesthetic preference and stress recovery. *Urban Forestry & Urban Greening, 41,* 6–13.

White Arkitekter. (2019). *Lindesberg Health Centre.* https://whitearkitekter.com/project/lindesberg-health-centre/

ZGF. (n.d.a). *Dana-Farber Cancer Institute, Yawkey Center for Cancer Care.* https://www.zgf.com/project/dana-farber-cancer-institute-yawkey-center-for-cancer-care/

ZGF. (n.d.b). *CHI Franciscan Health, St. Anthony Hospital Pendleton, OR* https://www.zgf.com/project/chi-franciscan-health-st-anthony-hospital/

ZGF. (n.d.c). *CHI Franciscan Health, St. Anthony Hospital Gig Harbor, WA* https://www.zgf.com/project/chi-franciscan-health-st-anthony-hospital-gigharbor/

9 Toward The Shifted Paradigms for Hospital Environment Design

This book examines the relationships between inside-out, architectural, and landscape spaces and people–nature transitions in large hospital environments through the lenses of patient-centered care and evidence-based design. Placing users' spatial experience in the center of the design process, this work proposed a preliminary pattern language of 12 transparent spaces that can be applied in healthcare design to enhance people–nature engagement in the public spaces of the hospital. Two recent experiments rigorously tested two dominant patterns that involve the fundamental forms of human–environment interactions: the "therapeutic viewing places" pattern concerns one's static status when resting, waiting, dining, or working in the hospital while the "transparent arteries" pattern emphasizes the importance of people's perceptions of and experiences with the hospital environment in motion. Experimental results indicated that large windows with quality views, abundant daylight, and a high level of transparency to gardens and nature calm people's stress, enhance their mood, and improve their spatial cognition and wayfinding; those transparency features are preferred, to a substantial extent, by people regarding the visual esthetics, attractiveness, and atmospheric pleasantness in large hospital environments.

Patient-Centered Care and User-Centered Design

Since the rise and spread of the patient-centered care concept in the 1990s, the respect for patients' experiences, preferences, and expressed needs have been advocated as being as critically important as the efficiency and efficacy of healthcare service delivery (Gerteis et al., 1993). The groundbreaking text *Through the Patients' Eyes: Understanding and Promoting Patient-Centered Care* outlined a conceptual framework that sheds light on seven dimensions of care for patients, among which several aspects are highly relevant to environmental design issues (Gerteis et al., 1993, pp. 5–11). Regarding the physical comfort dimension, "patients report heightened awareness of the cold, frightening, or gloomy institutional trappings of the hospital environment, and a parallel appreciation of clean, comfortable, and pleasant surroundings" (p. 8). Concerning the emotional and social support, family

DOI: 10.4324/9781003122180-9

and close friends were recognized as playing a central role in patients' experience of illness; therefore, the healthcare environmental design should accommodate the needs of families and friends to the greatest extent possible. The US Institute of Medicine (IOM) publication *Crossing the Quality Chasm* (2001) urged that patient care must be less provider-driven and more patient and family centered, with the patient's preferences, norms, and values respected. The design for the physical environments that organizes the delivery of healthcare services should follow the same approach that incorporates patients' preferences, beliefs, and values and includes patients' engagement in decision-making, known as patient-centered design (Stichler, 2011). Evaluating the outcomes of patient-centered care and design should embrace patients' and families' satisfaction with the healthcare experience, feelings of well-being, a sense of control and autonomy, involvement in care, engagement in a therapeutic relationship with care providers, and a sense of being in a healing and supportive environment (Stichler, 2011).

Through Patients' Eyes was published nearly 30 years ago, and many patient-centered approaches have since been integrated into institutional policies and facility guidelines that have significantly improved the quality and safety of care in large hospitals, yet challenges remain for the patient-centered agenda in continuing the current healthcare reformation (Groene, 2017). Some obvious gaps on the patient-centered agenda include, for instance, the care and support through environmental design for rapidly increased patient population with chronic conditions at the primary care level and more broadly in local communities (Groene, 2017). Many environmental designs that integrate high esthetics and state-of-the-art research evidence only exist in high-end facilities or elite organizations, and such differences in spatial qualities from community hospitals and clinics in rural areas are ever-expanding. The post-occupancy evaluations of healthcare environmental designs, defined as the process of evaluating buildings or landscape spaces in a systematic and rigorous manner after they have been built and occupied for some time from the perspective of occupants using the setting (Cooper Marcus & Francis, 1998; Preiser et al., 2015), are usually a link missing in the cycle of many healthcare projects.

A hospital facility cannot function without competent medical staff, nurses, and all sorts of supporting members. The hospital is a workplace relying on diverse employees, and many of them are traditionally considered to do offstage work. However, it is arguable that providing humanized work environments for all employees aligns with the optimal goal of a therapeutic hospital campus. One example is the shift in design trend from the centralized workstation for nurses to the decentralized nurse station and to the current hybrid model, which reflects the broadly inclusive, user-centered design concept in the current healthcare design. Decentralized nurse stations were claimed to enable nurses to provide better visual supervision of patients, reduce the noise level in the patient ward, and offer greater integration of information technology (McCullough, 2010). However, the trade-offs with centralized nurse stations are not negligible and include longer travel distances, isolation and inadequate socialization and collaboration during work, and disconnect from the outside (Zborowsky et al., 2010). In addition, the access to window views, daylight, and nature is significantly reduced in staff workplaces compared to patient rooms and public zones, and supporting staff such as facility managers and mechanical technicians often still work in windowless basements in even the best-designed hospitals. The elevated hospital environment and high design esthetics increase the sense of pride and work satisfaction among employees, which helps retain the medical care team and, in turn, provides positive care for patients. Therefore, following the broad user-centered design principles and offering universal opportunities for frequent person–nature encounters within the entire hospital campus are highly desired.

Integrating Evidence-Based Research and Design

The general public and patient populations frequently have contrasting esthetic preferences from designers. The types and styles of environmental design and art that many design professionals prefer can be those that elicit distinctly negative reactions from the public; several studies cited by Cooper Marcus and Barnes (1999) confirmed that patients consistently prefer nature-themed art and design styles over ambiguous and abstract art and features. Medical planners and designers should value the user advisory board and consult patients' opinions during each phase of the hospital design, ranging from the spatial layout at large to detailed interior decorations. However, the manipulated forms and spaces in architectural and landscape designs share significant overlaps with other forms of art through which the artists investigate the world through their own eyes, exclaim visual statements, and sway the viewers' opinions (Mesch, 2014). In such situations, evidence-based research and design (EBR&D) could play a role in reconciling the seemingly inherent conflicts between the designer-led and user-centered systems in healthcare design. A two-staged EBR&D framework has been proposed to integrate research inquiries into design and creativity by Verderber and colleagues (2014). The first stage embraces the long-standing intuitive model in art whereby creativity is fostered; in stage two, forecasting the performance of the conceptual design becomes the focus, whereby the use of multiple sources of knowledge is woven into design, followed by an intermediate post-design evaluation (Verderber et al., 2014). In a dynamic EBR&D cycle, meaningful research questions are generalizable from design intuition, and the design solutions are consistently refined through the quick testing of design concepts and the timely knowledge of transfer.

Contemporary technology has advanced rapidly to facilitate design simulations. Scale models and full-size cardboard mock-ups are thriving tools to aid with the testing of spatial design features (Joseph et al., 2017), and immersive virtual reality techniques (IVEs), offering high levels of immersion and flexibility in manipulating different variables, have become promising tools in the evaluation of healthcare design outcomes (Joseph et al., 2020). Inviting all stakeholders in multiple phases of the design process adds invaluable participatory design components that ensure the results meet the needs of different user groups. Up to this point, the evidence on which healthcare design relies should primarily come from empirical studies and scientific findings, then through careful consultancy with experts' knowledge bases and the critical review of users' direct input. The systematic documentation and publication of projects and the public sharing of research results that meet academic standards prepare references for future practices that achieve the ultimate Evidence-Based Design (EBD) mission (Hamilton, 2003).

The Shifting Paradigms of Hospital Environment Design

Since the 1990s, healthcare professionals in the US have been seeking design solutions to relieve the various environmental stressors in large hospitals, such as by using urban design strategies to guide medical planning and improve spatial orientation (Allison, 2007), decentralizing the mega-hospitals by redefining the functions in different buildings within a village-like campus (Verderber & Fine, 2000), and introducing nature and other positive distractions to hospital occupants for the overall stress reduction (Cooper Marcus & Sachs, 2013; Ulrich, 1999). Specifically, decentralizing hospital facilities differs from decentralizing the healthcare delivery system. The once cottage-like healthcare industry has deemed its inefficiency regarding the excessive costs of waste, inconsistent care quality and safety, and barriers to access and integrated information technology (Institute of Medicine, 2001). Meanwhile, the healthcare landscape is shifting toward clinical integration that improves multifaceted patient care in a more standardized manner (Devereux, n.d.). The once highly densified mega-hospitals are facing functional deconstruction, and hospital greenspaces could serve as nodes and hinges that connect and organize different functional zones.

The disconnect between architectural and landscape architectural spaces on a medical campus usually leads to unpleasant window views or inadequate usage of hospital gardens. In addition, the visibility and accessibility issues of many hospital gardens are also caused by the low priority of landscape design in the early phase of the master planning; suitable lands are too easily sacrificed for parking lots or other purposes. Hospital greenspaces are often seen as areas that separate buildings or that are left over, and the landscaped grounds may serve as "a reserve for future expansion of the healthcare facility and eventually be built over" (Cooper Marcus, 2007, p. 36). Influenced by the recent evidence-based design trends, many healthcare facilities have started implementing gardens by simply converting the existing, underutilized spaces on campus, but such a change barely makes a difference in the gloomy and depressing atmosphere in the deep center of

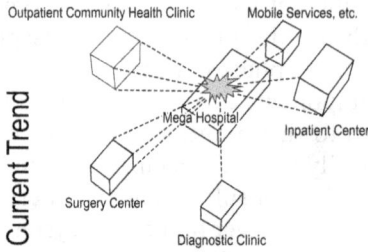

Functionally Deconstructed Mega-Hospital within a Campus (Verderber, 2010)

Image adapted from Clemson University_History of Healthcare Architecture_Spring 2006 http://courses.clemson.edu/dbattis-arch-885/modern.swf

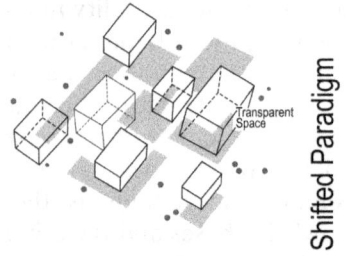

Windows, Transparency, and Integrative Therapeutic Landscapes in Large Hospitals

Image created by Jiang (2014)

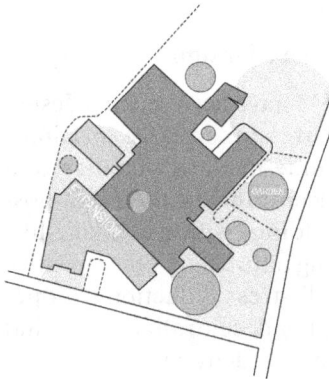

Current practices that integrate gardens on a medical campus but either in "leftover" spaces between building units or along the perimeter of the property, leaving the building interiors complicated in functions and circulations.

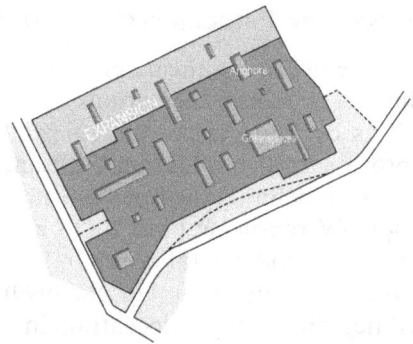

Shifted paradigm that strategically integrates multiple greenspaces in the building complex that provides wayfinding cues and positive distractions. Courtyards also serve as expansion links/anchors, connecting to a larger system of therapeutic landscapes

Figure 9.1 The current trend and shifting paradigms of hospital environment design

Source: Drawn by Shan Jiang and Udday Datta

the building mass, leaving a very small proportion of greenspaces compared to the overall square footage of the hospital interiors. The hospital buildings and campus should incorporate greenspaces and natural features that are visible, tangible, accessible, and memorable. Additional, gardens at key locations in the healthcare environment could serve as landmarks as well as the anchors for the future expansion of the facility. Therefore, new building components grow out of greenspaces and nature instead of the interior units that are already intricated spatially and functionally (Figure 9.1).

Roles of Landscape Architects

According to case studies on a series of healthcare design projects that demonstrated exemplary quality in landscape design, applying nature or park themes to guide the healthcare facility design generally forecasts delightful results, such as the "Institute in the Park" concept leading the design of the Alder Hey Children's hospital and its new research and education building (Liverpool, UK) and the Maggie's Cancer Caring Centre in Hong Kong, with the design being led by Frank Gehry, that arranged a series of six interconnected pavilions within a Chinese garden into which all rooms open to see the surrounding nature and ponds. Furthermore, landscape architects were found to play leadership roles starting in the early phases of the best practices that integrated landscape as an essential program element of the hospital design, help develop sustainable site development plans, arrange a hierarchical system of greenspaces, identify the most suitable locations for gardens, and coordinate indoor–outdoor connectivity throughout the campus. Summarized from a series of case studies documented by the Landscape Architecture Foundation (Jiang & Kaljevic, 2016a, 2016b, 2016c; Mattson & Guinn, 2013; Thoren & Louw, 2013), the roles the landscape architects could play in a healthcare design project are far more profound beyond the design of small garden pieces. Some additional roles include but are not limited to:

- Being an integral part of the design team that assesses the opportunities and constraints of the campus site and develops site design concepts that support the overall project goals, integrating landscape as an essential program of the hospital design
- Closely working with community groups and multiple stakeholders while being responsible for visioning and guiding the project toward design solutions that not only fulfill the needs of the owner and building program, but also establish a landscape that would be an amenity for local communities
- Assessing the needs of specific patient and family populations to create outdoor spaces responsive to their spiritual and psychological needs
- Developing native plant inventory and guidance on preserving the existing land and vegetation as well as developing a natural resource management and maintenance plan
- Developing plans for low-impact site development and stormwater management
- Coordinating multidisciplinary collaborations in the design and construction of the transitional spaces among architects, specialty engineers, lighting designers, and horticulturists

Trends of Hospital Greenspaces in the Pandemic Context

The COVID-19 pandemic will have a long-lasting impact on the health and life of the global population. It has already profoundly reshaped the healthcare systems and hospital facility designs in the US and many other countries. Experts have emphasized several key trends in the healthcare industry stemming from the pandemic, including telemedicine and hybrid experience, tailored patient engagement and precision medicine, prioritization of preventive care, and advocacy for equitable access to healthcare (Russell, 2021). Regarding the spatial design aspects of healthcare facilities, healing gardens and greenspaces could play innovative roles in the future hospitals, as summarized next.

Disappearing Waiting Rooms: Wait in a Garden!

Patients are able to schedule appointments through telemedicine portals, and fewer people will use waiting rooms in their future medical visits. For in-person visits during the pandemic, many patients were told to wait in their personal vehicles until being notified via a pager or text messages. In future hospital designs, planning waiting rooms adjacent to a courtyard or lightwell with operatable doors and windows will ensure greater flexibility when waiting; patients and family members could wait in a garden when weather allows it, enabling them to breathe fresh air while having a therapeutic experience. When the healthcare facility experiences an unusually high influx of patients, greenspaces adjacent to the waiting rooms could serve as a buffer and a triage area near the facility entrance.

Expanded Public Spaces with Integrated Nature Experience

Public spaces in future hospitals will require rapid expansion and subdivision, as needed, to accommodate social distancing and minimize the short-range transmission of virus. Integrating multiple courtyards and a variety of natural settings into the public spaces of a large healthcare facility could serve as nodes that divide functional units while accelerating natural ventilation. The balancing of contagion and connection has introduced new ethical dilemmas in healthcare delivery services in the pandemic context—namely, the isolation of confirmed infectious patients and the lack of human interactions yield significant mental and behavioral health risks (Anderson & Holmes, 2020). Views to the outside, daylight, and access to greenspaces make isolated patients feel that they are somewhat connected to the world, and sharing certain nature experiences among non-critical patients could help reestablish a social routine. Birthing and dying experiences should always allow for the option of loved ones being present at the first opportunity, and integrating temporary visiting pods that connect to the outdoor public spaces could allow for socially distanced connections (Anderson & Holmes, 2020; Cousins, 2020).

Hospital greenspaces serve essential functions, going beyond merely being looked at from the inside. Additional design suggestions for the hospital public spaces include shortening the typically long, narrow corridors and adding pocket gardens and breakout nooks along the circulation spaces to increase physical distancing. The avant-garde trend has further suggested using convertible partitions to enclose spaces; even the exterior wall can be movable, and the entire room could directly face and communicate with a garden outside. The removal of the needless walls could enable people to take shortcuts through free paths, thereby reducing traveling time inside the hospital building, which maximizes transportation efficiency and reduces the chance of virus infection. It could also break the arguably psychological boundary of glass and windows and extend people's nature experience beyond the pure visual dimension into a heightened experience that integrates haptic and sensory dimensions. The most direct interaction with nature—therapeutic gardening activities—has proven effective in treating many mental and physical conditions (Thompson, 2018) and should therefore also be strategically integrated in the current healthcare delivery system.

Gardens in Intensive Care Units

The COVID-19 pandemic revealed the shortage of intensive care units (ICUs) in many regions across the world, and it has become an imperative course to design more ICUs, or at least the flexible care units that can be easily transformed into ICUs, in the future hospital design. At the same time, there have been growing calls to return to the healing power of nature in ICUs for even the most critically ill patients (Verderber et al., 2021). Based on the latest evidence-based design guidelines, many ICUs have started including windows to introduce nature views and daylight in the patient bed areas (Thompson et al., 2012); preliminary research results have indicated significant stress-reducing effects among families and patients who take breaks in ICU gardens (Ulrich et al., 2020). Critical care professionals in the UK suggested integrating gardens as routine care in every ICU after seeing the clear therapeutic benefits of nature (Pugh, 2020). As part of a pioneering project at Derriford Hospital in Plymouth (Devon, UK), critical care patients—some still on ventilators—were sent outdoors for sunshine and fresh air to combat the virus. As described by an 84-year-old patient who survived COVID-19, the moment he felt the air on his face and saw the flowers after his bed was wheeled out into the ICU's "secret garden" was the "big breakthrough" in his recovery (Pugh, 2020). As this patient's recovery continued, he took part in basketball and skittles games with other COVID-19 patients in the garden. Other hospitals in London have started planning a roof garden in the ICU ward to help ill patients who have side effects such as delirium (Morris, 2020).

In addition, medical care providers and staff members in ICUs conduct complex treatments that follow more restrict routines, generally leading to a prevalence of high stress and severe burnout syndrome among them (Azoulay & Herridge, 2011; Kumar et al., 2016). During the COVID-19 pandemic, ICU staff members have faced the formidable challenge of infection threat, huge workloads and long-term fatigue, anxiety regarding unfamiliar working protocols, and frustration with the death of their patients (Shen et al., 2020). The integration of gardens and greenery in the most sophisticated and stressful unit in the hospital could provide an opportunity for a temporary "getaway" break.

Toward the Concept of Community Wellness Centers

During the pandemic, the spread of the disease and the implementation of governmental responses led to the increasing demand for park access worldwide, and some long-ignored benefits of greenspaces have been widely recognized by the public (Geng et al., 2021; Hockings et al., 2020). According to the *COVID-19 Community Mobility Reports* published by Google (n.d.), which show movement trends by region across different categories of places, the average increase of park visits from April 2020 to March 2021 was 13.9% for the entire US. when compared to the pre-pandemic baseline value. For example, in West Virginia, the state-level average increase of park visits during the one-year cycle of the pandemic (April 2020–March 2021) relative to baseline period was 30% (Society of Actuaries, n.d.). The planning and design of community open spaces and public natural resources for universal access and equitable use have become topical issues.

In the healthcare domain, there has been a rising call for the functional deconstruction of large hospital buildings and spread out the functional components across the local community (Verderber & Fine, 2000). The pandemic has revealed that the prevention of noncommunicable diseases has become an imperative action as the pandemic revealed the correlation between certain underlying medical conditions and the increased risk of severe illness from SARS-CoV-2 infection, including obesity, diabetes, cardiovascular disease, and more (Centers for Disease Control and Prevention, 2021). Two trends will stay strong in the post-pandemic era, including the community clinics that provide primary care and routine services, and microhospitals – small-scale inpatient facilities that offer wide-ranging medical services, often in underserved communities (Morgan & Burmahl, 2021). Some healthcare organizations and design professionals have suggested coining the community wellness center concept, which integrates walking trails, playgrounds, and therapeutic landscape features to support outdoor activities on the sites of a community clinic or microhospital. Some experimental programs to promote public health status, such as "walk with a doc," could be held in those greenspaces; healthcare professionals could have a conversation with the patient or conduct certain treatments outside, particularly for psychological and behavioral health patients. Such wellness centers aim not only to cure the sick but also to educate the public about active lifestyles and healthy diets, socialization and relationship bond, and disease prevention among residents in rural or medically underserved communities.

References

Allison, D. (2007). Hospital as city: Employing urban design strategies for effective wayfinding. *Health Facility Management, 20*(6), 61–65.

Anderson, D., & Holmes, M. (2020, December 17). How will COVID-19 change healthcare design?. *Design Museum Magazine, 17*, 68–75.

Azoulay, E., & Herridge, M. (2011). Understanding ICU staff burnout: The show must go on. *American Journal of Respiratory and Critical Care Medicine, 184*(10), 1099–2011. https://doi.org/10.1164/rccm.201109-1638ED

Centers for Disease Control and Prevention. (2021, May 13). COVID-19: People with certain medical conditions. https://www.cdc.gov/coronavirus/2019-ncov/need-extra-precautions/people-with-medical-conditions.html

Cooper Marcus, C. (2007). Healing gardens in hospitals. *Interdisciplinary Design and Research E-Journal, 1*(1).

Cooper Marcus, C., & Barnes, M. (Eds.). (1999). *Healing gardens: Therapeutic benefits and design recommendations* (Vol. 4). John Wiley & Sons.

Cooper Marcus, C., & Francis, C. (1998). *People places: Design guidelines for urban open space.* New Yok, NY: John Willey & Sons.

Cooper Marcus, C., & Sachs, N. A. (2013). *Therapeutic landscapes: An evidence-based approach to designing healing gardens and restorative outdoor spaces.* John Wiley & Sons.

Cousins, S. (2020, June 24). Rethink: How will Covid-19 affect healthcare design? *The RIBA Journal.* https://www.ribaj.com/intelligence/future-of-healthcare-design-in-post-pandemic-world

Devereux, S. (n.d.). *"Health villages"—Healthcare's new innovative response to integrated care-delivery challenges.* The Kinetix Group. https://thekinetixgroup.com/health-villages-healthcares-new-innovative-response-integrated-care-delivery-challenges/

Geng, D. C., Innes, J., Wu, W., & Wang, G. (2021). Impacts of COVID-19 pandemic on urban park visitation: A global analysis. *Journal of Forestry Research, 32*(2), 553–567.

Gerteis, M., Edgman-Levitan, S., Daley, J. et al. (Eds). (1993). *Through the patient's eyes: Understanding and promoting patient-centered care.* Jossey-Bass.

Google. (n.d.). *COVID-19 community mobility reports.* https://www.google.com/covid19/mobility/

Groene, O. (2017). Through the patient's eyes: 25 years of quality and safety research and the challenges ahead. *International Journal for Quality in Health Care, 29*(7), 887–888.

Hamilton, D. K. (2003). The four levels of evidence-based practice. *Healthcare Design, 3*(4), 18–26.

Hockings, M., Dudley, N., Elliott, W., Ferreira, M. N., Mackinnon, K., Pasha, M. K. S., & Chassot, O. (2020). Editorial essay: Covid-19 and protected and conserved areas. *Parks, 26*(1), 7–24.

Institute of Medicine, Committee on Quality of Health Care in America (2001, July 19). *Crossing the quality chasm: A new health system for the 21st century.* National Academies Press.

Jiang, S., & Kaljevic, S. (2016a). *Hennepin county Medical Center Whittier Clinic. Landscape performance series.* Landscape Architecture Foundation. https://doi.org/10.31353/cs1200

Jiang, S., & Kaljevic, S. (2016b). *Virtua Voorhees Hospital. Landscape performance series. Landscape performance series.* Landscape Architecture Foundation. https://doi.org/10.31353/cs1190

Jiang, S., & Kaljevic, S. (2016c). *Owensboro Health Regional Hospital. Landscape performance series. Landscape performance series.* Landscape Architecture Foundation. https://doi.org/10.31353/cs1210

Joseph, A., Browning, M. H., & Jiang, S. (2020). Using immersive virtual environments (IVEs) to conduct environmental design research: A primer and decision framework. *Health Environments Research & Design Journal, 13*(3), 11–25.

Joseph, A., Joshi, R., & Allison, D. (Eds.). (2017, May 1). *Realizing improved patient care through human-centered design in the operating room (RIPCHD.OR)* (Vol. 2). Center for Health Facilities Design & Testing, Clemson University. https://issuu.com/clemsonchfdt/docs/ripchd.or_vol._2

Kumar, A., Pore, P., Gupta, S., & Wani, A. O. (2016). Level of stress and its determinants among intensive care unit staff. *Indian Journal of Occupational and Environmental Medicine, 20*(3), 129.

Mattson, M. P., & Guinn, R. (2013). *Advocate Lutheran General Hospital Patient Tower. Landscape performance series.* Landscape Architecture Foundation. https://doi.org/10.31353/cs0560

McCullough, C. S. (Ed.). (2010). *Evidence-based design for healthcare facilities.* Sigma Theta Tau.

Mesch, C. (2014). *Art and politics: A small history of art for social change since 1945.* Bloomsbury Publishing.

Morgan, J., & Burmahl, B. (April 22, 2021). 2021 Hospital construction survey: Hospital and contractors take on pandemic-related building and design challenges. Health Facilities Management. https://www.hfmmagazine.com/articles/4148-2021-hospital-construction-survey

Morris, S. (May 5, 2020). Back to nature: "secret garden" outings used to aid coronavirus recovery. *The Guardian.* https://www.theguardian.com/world/2020/may/05/back-to-nature-secret-garden-outings-used-to-aid-coronavirus-recovery

Preiser, W. F., White, E., & Rabinowitz, H. (2015). *Post-occupancy evaluation* (Routledge Revivals). Routledge.

Pugh, R. (2020, May 22). *COVID-19: Therapeutic benefits of "secret" ICU gardens. Medscape.*

Russell, J. S. (2021, February 23). *What the post-pandemic hospital might look like.* Bloomberg CityLab. https://www.bloomberg.com/news/articles/2021-02-23/how-the-pandemic-is-transforming-hospital-design

Shen, X., Zou, X., Zhong, X., Yan, J., & Li, L. (2020). Psychological stress of ICU nurses in the time of COVID-19. *Critical Care, 24.* https://doi.org/10.1186/s13054-020-02926-2

Society of Actuaries. (n.d.). A tool for mapping and graphing Google's mobility dataset. https://www.soa.org/resources/research-reports/2020/google-mobility-data/

Stichler, J. F. (2011). Patient-centered healthcare design. *The Journal of Nursing Administration, 41*(12), 503–506.

Thompson, D. R., Hamilton, D. K., Cadenhead, C. D., Swoboda, S. M., Schwindel, S. M., Anderson, D. C., Schmitz, E. V., St. Andre, A. C., Axon, D. C., Harrell, J. W., Harvey, M. A., Howard, A., Kaufman, D. C., & Petersen, C. (2012). Guidelines for intensive care unit design. *Critical Care Medicine, 40*(5), 1586–1600.

Thompson, R. (2018). Gardening for health: A regular dose of gardening. *Clinical Medicine, 18*(3), 201–205.

Thoren, R., & Louw, A. (2013). *Randall Children's Hospital. Landscape performance series.* Landscape Architecture Foundation. https://doi.org/10.31353/cs0620

Ulrich, R. S. (1999). Effects of gardens on health outcomes: Theory and research. In C. Cooper Marcus, & M. Barnes (Eds.), *Healing gardens: Therapeutic benefits and design recommendations* (pp. 27–86). Wiley.

Ulrich, R. S., Cordoza, M., Gardiner, S. K., Manulik, B. J., Fitzpatrick, P. S., Hazen, T. M., & Perkins, R. S. (2020). ICU patient family stress recovery during breaks in a hospital garden and indoor environments. *Health Environments Research & Design Journal, 13*(2), 83–102.

Verderber, S., & Fine, D. J. (2000). *Healthcare architecture in an era of radical transformation.* Yale University Press.

Verderber, S., Gray, S., Suresh-Kumar, S., Kercz, D., & Parshuram, C. (2021). Intensive care unit built environments: A comprehensive literature review (2005–2020). *Health Environments Research & Design Journal.* https://doi.org/10.1177/19375867211009273

Verderber, S., Jiang, S., Hughes, G., & Xiao, Y. (2014). The evolving role of evidence-based research in healthcare facility design competitions. *Frontiers of Architectural Research, 3*(3), 238–249.

Zborowsky, T., Bunker-Hellmich, L., Morelli, A., & O'Neill, M. (2010). Centralized vs. decentralized nursing stations: Effects on nurses' functional use of space and work environment. *Health Environments Research & Design Journal, 3*(4), 19–42.

Index

Note: Page numbers in bold refer to tables; those followed by 'n' refer to notes.

For Product Safety Concerns and Information please contact our EU
representative GPSR@taylorandfrancis.com
Taylor & Francis Verlag GmbH, Kaufingerstraße 24, 80331 München, Germany